Nursing Theories
in Practice

Nursing Theories in Practice

Marilyn E. Parker, Editor

Pub. No. 15-2350

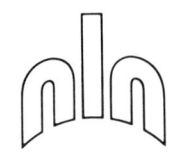

National League for Nursing

Copyright © 1990
National League for Nursing
350 Hudson Street, New York, NY 10014

All rights reserved. No part of this book may be reproduced in print, or by photostatic means, or in any other manner, without the express written permission of the publisher.

ISBN 0-88737-497-2

> The views expressed in this publication represent the views of the authors and do not necessarily reflect the official views of the National League for Nursing.

This book was set in Garamond and Goudy by Publications Development Company. The editor and designer was Rachel Schaperow. Northeastern Press was the printer and binder. The cover was designed by Lillian Welsh.

Reprint 2.0M-0892-025950

Printed in the United States of America

Contents

Contributors ix

Preface xiii

PART 1: Introduction

1. **Developing Perspectives on Nursing Theory in Practice** 3
   Marilyn E. Parker

2. **Nurses' Responses to the Nursing Theorist Conferences** 7
   Savina O. Schoenhofer

3. **Reflecting a Vision** 13
   Fay Gardner

PART 2: Johnson's Behavioral System Model for Nursing

4. **The Behavioral System Model for Nursing** 23
   Dorothy E. Johnson

5. **Implementation of the Johnson Model: One Hospital's Experience** 33
   Vivien Dee

PART 3: Orem's Self-Care Deficit Theory of Nursing

6. A Nursing Practice Theory in Three Parts, 1956–1989   47
   Dorothea E. Orem

7. Practical Applications of Orem's Self-Care Deficit Nursing Theory   61
   Susan G. Taylor

PART 4: King's Theory of Goal Attainment

8. King's Conceptual Framework and Theory of Goal Attainment   73
   Imogene M. King

9. Implementing King's Conceptual Framework at the Bedside   85
   Esther Byrne Coker and Rita Schreiber

PART 5: Martha Rogers' Theoretical Framework for Nursing

10. Space-Age Paradigm for New Frontiers in Nursing   105
    Martha E. Rogers

11. Practical Application of Rogers' Theoretical Framework for Nursing   115
    Linda Joseph

PART 6: Newman's Theory of Health

12. Shifting to Higher Consciousness   129
    Margaret A. Newman

13. Application of Newman's Theory of Health: Pattern Recognition as Nursing Practice   141
    Winnifred Gustafson

14. The Gift: Applying Newman's Theory of Health in Nursing Practice   163
    Kathleen A. Kalb

PART 7: Levine's Conservation Model

15. **Conservation and Integrity**   189
    Myra E. Levine

16. **Application of Levine's Conservation Model to Nursing the Homeless Community**   203
    Jane B. Pond

17. **A Description of Fatigue Associated with Congestive Heart Failure: Use of Levine's Conservation Model**   217
    Karen Moore Schaefer

PART 8: The Neuman Systems Model

18. **The Neuman Systems Model: A Theory for Practice**   241
    Betty M. Neuman

19. **Implementation of the Neuman Systems Model in an Acute Care Nursing Department**   263
    Margaret M. Moynihan

PART 9: Watson's Theory of Caring in Nursing

20. **Transpersonal Caring: A Transcendent View of Person, Health, and Healing**   277
    M. Jean Watson

21. **Watson's Theory of Caring in Nursing: The Rainbow of and for People Living with AIDS**   289
    Ruth M. Neil

Contributors

Esther Byrne Coker, MScN, RN
Clinical Education Specialist
Chedoke-McMaster Hospitals
Hamilton, Ontario, Canada

Vivien Dee, DNSc, CNAA, RN
Associate Hospital Administrator, Director of Nursing
UCLA Neuropsychiatric Institute and Hospital
Assistant Dean, Clinical Affairs
UCLA School of Nursing
Los Angeles, California

Fay Gardner, MSN, RN
Director of Education
Cedars Medical Center
Miami, Florida

Winnifred Gustafson, MS, RN
Parish Nurse, Gloria Dei Lutheran Church
Duluth, Minnesota

Dorothy E. Johnson, MPH, RN
Professor Emerita
University of California Los Angeles
School of Nursing
Los Angeles, California

Linda Joseph, BSN, RN
Graduate Student in Nursing
Florida Atlantic University
Boca Raton, Florida

Kathleen A. Kalb, RNC
PhD Candidate
Perinatal Clinical Nurse Specialist
Abbott Northwestern Hospital
Minneapolis, Minnesota

Imogene M. King, EdD, RN
Professor of Nursing
University of South Florida
Tampa, Florida

Myra E. Levine, MSN, RN, FAAN
Professor Emerita
College of Nursing
University of Illinois at Chicago
Chicago, Illinois

Margaret M. Moynihan, MS, RN
Assistant Director of Nursing
Mount Sinai Hospital
Hartford, Connecticut

Ruth M. Neil, MN, RN
PhD Candidate
Project Director, Denver Nursing Project in Human Caring
University of Colorado School of Nursing
Denver, Colorado

Betty M. Neuman, PhD, RN
Independent Practice
Beverly, Ohio

Margaret A. Newman, PhD, RN, FAAN
Professor
School of Nursing
University of Minnesota
Minneapolis, Minnesota

Dorothea E. Orem, BSNed, MSNed
Consultant in Nursing
Savannah, Georgia

Marilyn E. Parker, PhD, RN
Assistant Professor of Nursing
Florida Atlantic University
Boca Raton, Florida

Jane B. Pond, MSN, RNC, CRNP
Nursing Director, Homeless Programs
Philadelphia Health Management Corporation
Philadelphia, Pennsylvania

Martha E. Rogers, ScD, RN, FAAN
Professor Emerita
The Division of Nursing
New York University
New York, New York

Karen Moore Schaefer, DNSc, RN
Associate Professor
Allentown College of St. Francis de Sales
Center Valley, Pennsylvania
Nurse Researcher
The Allentown Hospital–Lehigh Valley Hospital Center
Allentown, Pennsylvania

Savina O. Schoenhofer, PhD, RN
Associate Professor of Nursing
Graduate Program Director
Florida Atlantic University
Boca Raton, Florida

Rita Schreiber, MS, RN,
Clinical Nurse Specialist
Queen Street Mental Health Center
Toronto, Ontario, Canada

Susan G. Taylor, PhD, RN
Associate Professor of Nursing
University of Missouri-Columbia
Columbia, Missouri

M. Jean Watson, PhD, RN, FAAN
Dean and Professor, School of Nursing
Director, Center for Human Caring
University of Colorado Health Sciences Center
Denver, Colorado

Preface

This book presents the most recent explications of major nursing theories and offers rich descriptions of the use of these theories in nursing practice. Contributors to this book are nurses who were invited to present their work at the South Florida Nursing Theorist Conferences sponsored by Cedars Medical Center, Miami, in spring 1989 and spring 1990. This book, and the conferences, are directed to nurses concerned with relating nursing theory to practice. It is hoped that this book will enrich both the theory and the practice of nursing and in so doing will adequately reflect the intention behind the conferences.

Each chapter in this book is an original work prepared for presentation at one of the conferences and for inclusion in this book. Chapters prepared by nursing theorists include current thinking beyond that presented in previously published work. The contributions by nurses about their use of theory in practice leave no doubt of the value of nursing theory to nursing practice. Three introductory chapters offer insight into the development of the theories conferences, responses of nurses attending the conferences, and perspectives on the use of nursing theory that emerged from the conferences. Two major presenters are not included in this volume because they chose to publish their work elsewhere.

The arrangement of chapters in this book follows the format of the conferences: each major theorist preceded a nurse or nurses who discussed the use of the theory in her (or their) practice or in a practice setting. Many contributors have extended their verbal presentations in written form. Many authors retained the use of first person as a means to enhance personal expression and permit the reader a closer acquaintance with the writer. This reflects the mood of the conferences, in which the presenters actively participated in the conference with other nurses. The wide variety of practice situations where nursing theory is explicitly used is exciting, and the use of nursing theory in nursing administration presents encouraging possibilities for facilitating the use of nursing theory in practice.

The stimulus for these conferences came from nurses at Cedars Medical Center. It has been noted how appropriate it is that nursing theories conferences focused on practice originated in a nursing service setting. Fay Gardner of Cedars provided the vision and leadership for these conferences. Her vision and leadership were confirmed as nurses in various roles in practice, administration, education, and scholarship came together at the conferences to help make her vision live. The response and active enthusiasm of each presenter and each participant was immediate, genuine, and continuing.

The encouragement and help of Sally J. Barhydt, Managing Editor at the National League for Nursing, to acclaim the importance of this work by its publication assures that many nurses will benefit from these endeavors. The careful editing by Rachel Schaperow of the Communications Division of the National League for Nursing has provided a consistently readable set of chapters. All of us are grateful for the skill, commitment, and cooperation of Sally and Rachel. All proceeds from the sale of this book will benefit future efforts toward the use of nursing theories in practice at Cedars Medical Center.

Marilyn E. Parker, PhD, RN
West Palm Beach, Florida
June 1990

Part 1

Introduction

1

Developing Perspectives on Nursing Theory in Practice

Marilyn E. Parker

The main objective of the two South Florida Nursing Theorist Conferences was to enhance the meaning of nursing theory for nursing practice. The intention was to assist nurses to make theory live in practice and thus enrich both nursing theory and practice. Readiness for these outcomes soon became apparent. The conferences were highlighted by the opportunity to ask questions about nursing theory and its usefulness, about development and evaluation of nursing theory, and about the nurses who develop and use the theories. Participants gathered with theorists and those who shared their use of nursing theory to explore theories and applications, get to know each other in personal and collegial ways, and begin to evolve possibilities together. Relations between nursing theory and nursing practice were uncovered and illuminated.

Some of the perspectives on nursing theories that evolved during the conferences will be introduced in this chapter in the hope that nurses reading the following chapters will benefit from work to discover ways to use nursing theory toward knowing and creating solutions.

Our day-to-day professional lives seem to be directed by diagnostic related groupings, measures of patient acuity, quality statements, and measures of this quality. We face issues of flexible staffing, cost effectiveness, educational advancement, retention, recruitment, image, professionalism, and autonomy. We feel thrust into management and economics to the neglect of the nursing of our patients and clients. We fear that clinical nursing will increasingly take a backseat to the requirements of reporting and recording. Our anchor in the sea of issues and problems is an explicit conception of nursing, knowledge of nursing theory, and the use of nursing theory in practice, administration, education, and scholarship.

In order to use theory we must think, question, discuss, study, explore, take risks, and by so doing realize our caring and commitment to nursing and our nurse colleagues. Nursing theories are designed for various purposes and are developed on various levels. They must be evaluated in order to determine their usefulness. To use a nursing theory is not to apply it *onto* a nursing situation but rather to see that the theory is embodied in, and is inseparable from, the fabric of the situation. To understand and employ nursing theory is a challenge. The asking of questions may assist in making nursing theory more available and usable to nurses in practice.

QUESTIONS ABOUT NURSING THEORY AND PRACTICE

Nurses may begin to think about the application of nursing theory to practice by asking the following questions: What is the meaning of nursing to me? What is my definition of nursing? What concepts represent my mental view of nursing? What do I do with my patients? Why do I do it, and what do I hope to achieve by my nursing actions? What is special, valuable, and unique about nursing? Such questions help us learn about ourselves as nurses and about our interactions as we serve others. From such a basis, we can continue to question and thus come to understand our conceptualization of nursing.

What is nursing theory? What makes a theory a nursing theory? What is not a nursing theory? What theories are used in nursing that are not nursing theories? How are various nursing theories and other theories related?

We may ask these questions in regard to each theory we contemplate using. What is the nursing focus of the theory and is this consistent with nursing as I know it? Can this theory provide guidance in many nursing practice situations? Is this theory so general that it will fit any helping situation or so specific that only selected areas of practice are appropriate for its use? In what ways will this theory help my nursing practice? What will it do and what will it not do for me? What can I contribute to this theory and its application through my work in nursing practice?

How can each one of us approach the challenge to understand and use nursing theory? In what ways can we encourage ourselves and other nurses to explore new views of nursing and perhaps further the development of nursing as a discipline and a professional practice? What are our resources? What are our tools?

DEVELOPING PERSPECTIVES THROUGH KNOWING OTHER NURSES

Discussing nursing with those who develop and use nursing theory provides another way to develop perspectives on nursing theories and their uses. The spirit of community that comes from the recognition that nursing scholars and nursing practitioners share the same understandings and dreams for nursing can be expressed as gratitude for richer and more complete knowing.

Goodness and hope can be recognized in nursing theory. The nursing theorists have shared their creative work in writing and speaking, and they have shared themselves at the conferences so that many nurses are now better acquainted with them. These theorists have contributed to an increased sense of unity in nursing.

Each nursing theorist who has so honored nursing and nurses began the work of theory development during years when few nurses knew, understood, or cared for their goals and efforts. They demonstrated vision, courage, and a love of nursing with relatively little support or encouragement. Their belief in the value of nursing and their hope for its future carried them through many dry times.

Many of the present generation of nurses engaged in practice and research recognize that nursing theory is perhaps the best answer to the problems and challenges of the future of our discipline. Today we are willing and anxious to engage with nursing theorists, to contribute to their work through our practice, research, and our own development of theory. All members of our discipline may claim representation by those who attended the theorist conferences and may join us in expressing gratitude to the theorists of nursing.

The nurses who shared their applications of nursing theories at the conferences demonstrated the practicality of nursing theory and have thus helped us to realize important lessons. One of these lessons is that each of us uses nursing concepts and theories daily to guide our nursing actions. When we encounter a difficulty, we immediately survey and select concepts to help us deal with the challenge. The constructs in our minds frame and direct our practice.

The second lesson comes from the variety of applications of nursing theories and reminds us that each of us has unique talents, interests, and values. Our individual attributes result in a variety of world views that guide us in selecting and using theoretical formulations. We can also conclude that not every theory is for use by every nurse, but that theory is definitely effective for nursing. We select and use theories as individual nurses.

Gratitude is due each nurse who participated in the conferences. Many nurses have shown that they will no longer be satisfied to only notice and give scant attention to nursing theory. It is no longer acceptable to these nurses to view nursing theory as lofty and impractical. Participants at these conferences have recognized that there is a bond between nursing theory and practice that must be strengthened and nourished. Nursing theorists have known this for many years; each year theory becomes more real for more nurses. The challenge belongs to all nurses to move this knowing forward.

2

Nurses' Responses to the Nursing Theorist Conferences

Savina O. Schoenhofer

Nursing theory is considered to be of great interest and relevance to academicians in nursing. Practicing nurses, prepared at an entry level with no further formal nursing education, are either bored or overwhelmed with the idea of nursing theory—or so conventional wisdom would have it. Bedside nurses, floor nurses, nurses "in the trenches" only want the "how to's" and are quite content to leave the finer points of the discipline to those in ivory towers or front offices. Many people would agree with this point of view.

Data drawn from evaluations of the South Florida Nursing Theorist Conferences, held in 1989 and 1990, contradict this concept of who is interested in nursing theory and why. Einstein is credited with saying that there is nothing so practical as a good theory, and our data indicate this is so.

Of the more than 200 nurses attending the 1989 conference and completing the evaluation questionnaire, 41 percent worked in clinical practice and another 24 percent worked in nursing service administration, totaling 65 percent in applied settings. In response to the question, "will you have an opportunity to apply information from this conference in your practice?" 151 nurses

(88 percent) said "yes." Respondents were invited to write in comments describing an important lesson they learned at the conference, and 81 percent made the effort to do so.

As a prelude to analyzing and summarizing nurses' expressions of the meaning of their experiences with nursing and with nursing theorists at the conference, I wanted to try to articulate the meaning of the conference to me. Reflecting on the entire experience of daring to plan, witnessing the program and its impact, and then planning anew for the next conference, the meaning for me emerged clearly. We came together to honor and celebrate the discipline of nursing. The themes expressed in the conference evaluations reflected this feeling as well.

Simply understood, the idea of a discipline calls to mind a way of life, of being, of living. Nurses' expressions of their experiences communicated deeply held values, reflecting nursing not merely as a science, devoid of value, but as an ontology, a living of values.

King and Brownell's (1966) characteristics of disciplines provide a framework for illuminating meanings nurses gave to these experiences of honoring and celebrating the discipline of nursing. In addition to comments drawn from conference evaluation forms, ideas expressed by presenters have been incorporated to enhance this summary of the meaning of these conferences to the participants.

COMMUNITY OF SCHOLARS

A discipline is, first and foremost, a community of scholars (King & Brownell, 1966). This characteristic encompasses a wealth of meanings—persons unified in their love of an important idea, freedom of thought and expression within this unity, tradition and possibility, avenues for maintaining connectedness. The sense of community is perhaps the most palpable feature of these conferences. Martha Rogers said it first: "Nursing is a learned profession." A learned profession is a collective of persons with a shared vision, a shared mission, and a shared commitment to developing and expressing both vision and mission.

On one evaluation form, a head nurse reflected, "nursing theory in practice could help with current conflicts in nursing, eg.

DRGs, documentation." "Nursing theory must be administratively supported and encouraged; administrators need knowledge of the discipline of nursing," a director of nursing service wrote. A nurse in a staff development role wrote, "theory-based practice provides the essential basis for professional practice."

A staff nurse wrote that she learned at the conference the importance of "understanding others' ways of living, feeling, doing." Peg Moynihan said nursing theory "helps me reconstruct what we have done in nursing." Karen Schaefer acknowledged, "we don't all see things the same way—multiple models enable us to accommodate that." An inservice educator wrote, "we all have the same thoughts on what nursing is—our expression of nursing, however, is represented by different theories." A faculty member wrote, "let us thrive on our differences, not be threatened by them."

Membership in a community of scholars was evident among participants in these nursing theorist conferences. A clinical specialist expressed her respect for the various roles that contribute to our shared mission: "I loved meeting the theorists (kind of like meeting Elijah and St. Peter), but the practical application was the best part." One diploma graduate, a head nurse, noted "it was enlightening to be in a roomful of nurses, and all of them were positive about advancing nursing and the nursing image." A faculty member shared a renewed commitment, writing that the conference offered an opportunity to learn "from noted theorists I had not thought to meet in a lifetime—what a dream to behold . . . [the conference] increased my horizon to think of what *I* can do for the nursing profession." An inservice educator wrote that this is the "best of times to be a nurse." Finally, referring to the homeless, but with relevance also for nursing as a discipline, Jane Pond pointed out that "the challenge of the nurse is to find the community."

DOMAIN, WITH SUBSTANTIVE AND SYNTACTICAL STRUCTURE

A discipline represents a specified area of focus, contains knowledge organized to accomplish the purposes of the discipline, and generates rules that guide the activities of the discipline (King &

Brownell, 1966). These characteristics express the values, goals, and activities of the community of scholars making up the discipline. The very purpose of the South Florida Nursing Theorist Conferences is to bring to all nurses a full awareness of the work of members of the practice discipline to discover, create, and articulate current understandings of the domain and substantive and syntactical structure of nursing.

Myra Levine said that "to bring together the best science and the most devoted humanism is the ultimate aim of nursing." Betty Neuman made reference to a profession within a profession, "We'll be able to tell others what we are doing and why." A master's-prepared nurse administrator noted that "we can only see what we have a theory about." The importance of using "frameworks and theories to help us answer the question of 'what is nursing?'" was a lesson identified by one clinical specialist. An important lesson for one staff developer was the fact of "derivation of theory from differing paradigms." A staff nurse prepared with an associate degree commented, "nursing as a profession will require multiple nursing models."

An advanced registered nurse practitioner wrote, "theory application is of utmost importance if nursing is to progress as a unified science." A staff nurse wrote of the "need to move away from the medical model, toward a unique nursing model;" she added, "there is hope for nursing."

Donna Campbell, the chief nursing service administrator at Cedars, acknowledged that "nursing theory grounds nursing executives in the reality of nursing." Finally, as only a staff nurse could say it, the conference was "very interesting for an older RN with no knowledge or background in theory—there is more to nursing than mechanics!"

AN EXPRESSION OF HUMAN IMAGINATION

A discipline is a medium through which the fullness of being human can be illuminated. All of the hopes and dreams, joys and sorrows, thrills and frustrations that are a part of the human experience are lived in the context of a discipline (King & Brownell, 1966). That nursing as a discipline is an expression of human imagination is clearly borne out in the tone poems and word pictures created in response to the conference evaluation form.

Margaret Newman, in discussing the use of nursing theory, invited nurses to "put themselves into it and be creative with it." Karen Schaefer recognized the dynamic nature of nursing theory, noting that "the theorists are constantly evolving their models." A staff nurse commented "we need to be visionary in conceptualizing nursing."

Rather than obscuring the essence of nursing, participants found that the conference clarified and strengthened this essence. "Caring for the client is the main concern" emerged as an important theme of the conference for one nurse. Another discovered that "nursing is interpersonal, not behavioral." A nurse practitioner realized "that the nurse is affected by all interactions as well as the patient." A staff nurse with associate degree preparation commented, "attending [the conference was] like a fresh breeze blowing into my 25 years of nursing—it renewed my thinking toward the quality and how we can contribute more to the client as we advance in nursing in the 90s."

The depth of involvement experienced by nurses coming together from all walks of nursing life is represented in the following excerpts. A master's degree nursing student suggested that "theory-based practice may increase nurses' self-esteem." A staff nurse wrote that participation in the nursing theorist conference has "renewed my interest in nursing—I have a new sense of direction." Another staff nurse responded similarly, "[the conference] revitalized my feeling of nursing . . . I'm excited to see the future with use of nursing theory in practice." A clinical specialist wrote, "thank you for the opportunity to experience pride in my profession." Involvement in a community of scholars experiencing nursing theory moved one staff nurse to express the meaning of these conferences in this way: "let go . . . let flow . . . hope . . . goodness . . . love for my beloved profession."

REFERENCE

King, A., & Brownell, J. (1966). *The curriculum and the disciplines of knowledge.* New York: John Wiley & Sons.

3

Reflecting a Vision

Fay Gardner

The vision I have of nursing becoming a profession is beginning to be realized. I believe theory-based practice defines the uniqueness of nursing and validates the profession as a legitimate science and art. Theory-based practice is, as Susan Taylor said at the 1989 conference, "not simple or common sense," and is not just for scholars but for every practicing nurse. The Nursing Theorist Conferences at Cedars Medical Center have opened the eyes of many practicing nurses to an array of nursing theories and their clinical applications. Knowledge of these theories will allow nurses to choose a framework which best fits their practice.

I have been asked to tell you the story of my journey to this point. It has been long and circuitous, but the inspiration to develop a nursing philosophy while at Teachers College and the challenge to move nursing forward to become a profession, have been the focus of my life's work. I am in my stride in life, educating, taking others from where they are in their lives to a juncture where they can begin to consider the possibilities of what the nursing

---

Note: This paper was prepared with the assistance of Charlotte Barry and Cathie Wallace, graduate students in the School of Nursing, Florida Atlantic University, Boca Raton, Florida.

discipline can be. Reflecting on my life and how I've come to be what I am, it is difficult for me to relate how the choices I've made have become opportunities for growth. I hope reading my story will help you as your own journey and visions unfold.

I grew up in Jamaica, the youngest of nine children in a loving family. From the beginning, my parents emphasized the power of faith and the importance of education—principles which would give me direction in life. It was in this atmosphere of support and encouragement that I completed high school and entered training to become a nurse. After receiving my diploma at Kingston Public Hospital in Jamaica, I went on to study midwifery in England. During these studies in London I heard the call to teach nursing. As a certified nurse midwife, I was terribly disappointed to discover that, at age 24, I was too young to be an instructor in England. This disappointment temporarily dashed my hopes of teaching, and I made an immediate decision to return home to Jamaica. I didn't know then that this choice would open up a much broader horizon to me.

My journey home from London took me through New York City, where my studies for my bachelor's and master's degrees began rather serendipitously. I visited my oldest sister seeking consolation, but received instead the inspiration to return to school at Columbia University Teachers College. I applied as an exchange student, took comprehensive exams, received credit for previous educational experiences, and was admitted with advanced standing. Under the counsel of two professors there, Mildred Montag and Eleanor Lambertson, I became empowered with possibilities for myself and for nursing. Lambertson, my initial academic advisor, not only guided my program of study but became my mentor. Mildred Montag, a prime mover in the community college concept in the United States, was my first professor. As a student in her class, I turned in what I believed was a fine research paper, only to receive it back with many comments and suggestions in red. The hard thinking that followed this experience changed how I approached the rest of my work at Teachers College. I don't think Montag realized how she affected my life by that paper, but after that, I knew challenges could be faced and met.

Completing my bachelor's and master's degrees took two full years of carrying a maximum course load each term. As an undergraduate student, I was introduced to the works of early nurse scholars: Virginia Henderson, Hildegard Peplau, and Dorothea Orem. Their works, combined with the visionary concepts of Martha Rogers, became the foundation for my own developing philosophy of nursing. Throughout my graduate work, I came to know that nursing curricula should be built on philosophic beliefs about person, society, nursing, and the teaching-learning process. For my thesis, I developed a four-year, value-based curriculum that was adapted from a university on Long Island, New York. My ambition was to take this concept of philosophy-based nursing curricula home to Jamaica. However, Margaret Adams, my master's program advisor, cautioned the curriculum might not be transplantable. She encouraged me to consider cultural differences and the need to temper my thinking with that of nursing leadership in Jamaica.

Besides providing the chance to grow in my nursing education, the three years I spent in New York City allowed me to become reacquainted with a friend from Jamaica. Keith Gardner was studying at the University of Nebraska, but would come to visit relatives in New York City on vacations. We fell in love and were married before I completed my thesis. We have raised three children, sharing responsibilities for their care as we pursued our own professional development. While growing up, our children would ask, "Mommy, why at night, when we call, only Daddy comes?" He never woke me unless they had a fever he could not break. Just as he sustains me in our family life, he is always behind me in my commitment to nursing as my life's work.

After receiving my degrees, we returned to Jamaica where I was instrumental in developing a curriculum based on a synthesis of the conceptual models of Henderson and Orem for the University Hospital of the West Indies School of Nursing. At the same time, nursing education in Jamaica was changing dramatically. Basic hospital training was being replaced by a program where nurse trainees had student status, were given instruction in classrooms, and were taken into clinical areas for supervised practice. These changes paralleled the movement in the United States where hospital-based nurse training programs were progressing toward collegiate education for nurses. This was the most innovative change in nursing education since Nightingale's founding of the St. Thomas Hospital Training School for Nursing in 1860.

My commitment to the profession and my idea of professionalism being grounded in education led me back to Teachers College in 1968 to pursue a doctoral degree. There I looked at my own philosophy of nursing and how conceptual models could provide the structure for nursing practice. Challenged once again by the academia at Teachers College, my role in raising nursing to professional status became clearer. I became energized with the notion that as an educator, I could facilitate this ideal for nursing practice. My belief then, as well as now, is that nursing has its own theoretical body of knowledge that continually grows, changes, and evolves through the efforts of nurse researchers, educators, and practitioners. The commitment to practice from this knowledge base will bring nursing forward to professional status. In the 1960s, I thought nursing would become a profession within 20 years, but changes come slowly. By exposing nurses to different conceptual models for practice, their eyes can be opened to new possibilities. Courage is needed to allow the nursing profession to unfold in its own way, and patience is needed to allow it to grow in its own time.

Without finishing my doctoral studies, I returned home to Jamaica to be with my husband and young children. My vision of nursing as a profession stayed with me as I began working for the government, organizing a practical nurse training program and reinstituting a psychiatric nursing program. In the late 1970s, I was invited by the Jamaican Minister of Health to enroll in the University of Wisconsin pediatric nurse practitioner program. I saw this expanded practitioner role and its potential for autonomous practice as another step closer to professionalism for nursing. It was at Wisconsin that Nancy Diekelmann, assistant professor at the School of Nursing, took my class through the formation and development of a conceptual framework. This exercise brought me up to date with current advances in theory development and became my springboard for looking at newly developing nursing theories.

Having completed the nurse practitioner program in six months I again returned to Jamaica, filled with new knowledge and enthusiasm for establishing the first pediatric and family nurse practitioner programs in the country. One year after initiating the programs, my husband and I decided to leave Jamaica, this time probably for good. Our son needed special education unavailable in Jamaica. Through talking with others about our son's needs, I felt a strong intuitive sense that Miami was the right place for us to be. We made the move to Miami.

In 1980, I became a nurse educator at Cedars Medical Center. The following year, the nursing education department made a decision to include informal half hour sessions about nursing theory in the nursing orientation. Since most nurses had not been exposed to the idea of nursing theory, our effort was directed toward increasing their awareness about theories. Because of my background, I became a resource for theory information, providing articles and reference materials about specific theorists or nursing models. I planted seeds of theory-based practice as a means to professionalism and hoped they would take hold.

I was further stimulated to bring nursing theory to the practicing nurse after hearing Imogene King at a Miami workshop for educators in 1983. Nurses at that conference expressed a tremendous interest in learning more about theory and how it could provide structure and form for their practice. I imagined then hosting a nursing theorist conference by 1988, where several theories would be presented.

In my new role as Assistant Director of Nursing Education, I kept this dream in the back of my mind as my energies focused on motivating Cedars' nurses to continue their education. The first step was to set the stage. I began talking with each nurse for half an hour during orientation about educational opportunities available. I asked, "Now that you're here at Cedars, what are you doing with your nursing life?" At first, few were involved in any kind of scholarly study, so it has been very rewarding to see so many return to school. A strong educational foundation at the baccalaureate level will provide the footholds on which the profession can build. At Cedars we recognize the difference of practice based on education and compensate nurses for their advanced degrees and practice. There still exists much resistance to seeking higher degrees in nursing, so new ways must be found to encourage nurses to expand their knowledge, thus creating infinite possibilities for them as their lives unfold.

Our continual promotion of education for Cedars' nurses, coupled with the seeds I planted about theory-based practice, formed a favorable climate for the planning of the first theorist conference. An essential component of the process was waiting until the timing was right before involving key people. Fortune's favors abounded when I approached the Vice President of Nursing Services, Donna Campbell, with my program proposal. She immediately supported hosting a Nursing Theorist Conference at Cedars, believing this would remove the academic aura that traditionally surrounds theory. Administration, represented initially by Elly Howard, Vice President of Human Resources, endorsed the plan without reservations. The final approval was given by the President and Chief Executive Officer, Daniel Stickler, who vigorously promotes living of the hospital mission statement, encouraging continued education as the key to insure excellence in nursing care and services.

The next step was to invite nurse educators from area universities, colleges, and hospitals to join a think tank committee. The response was astounding, with educators from Barry University, Florida Atlantic University, Miami Dade Community College, University of Miami, and Baptist Hospital comprising the initial planning committee. Ideas flowed freely as we planned the conference. Within six months, the program was organized around the theme "Using Nursing Theory in Clinical Practice," objectives were developed, and speakers were confirmed.

During our think tank sessions, we planned the program format. Each nurse theorist presenting would be followed by a description of an actual practical application of the theory. This format was based on our using the word "practical" as meaning "related to practice." Our belief was that the practice exemplars would make the theories real by demonstrating their use in every day nursing situations. The concept was unique for this geographical area, as all prior area theory conferences focused on one or more theorists presenting their ideas without any corroborative practical applications of the theories. The suggestion to organize a poster session for displaying further clinical applications of the presenters' theories also arose from the think tank process.

The overwhelming positive response to the first conference and the desire for more exposure to nursing theorists by staff nurses led to the decision to hold a second conference in April 1990. This session was attended by a higher percentage of staff nurses from our community, validating our belief that we presented useful information for the practicing nurse. Graduate students from Florida Atlantic University organized a colloquium held at the close of the second conference. This gathering of theorists, practical application presenters, professors, students, and other practicing nurses met to discuss nursing. After hearing this dialogue and reading the conference evaluations, I know the thinking of nurses is changing. This provides the momentum to plan for theorists to meet with us again in the spring of 1991.

Exploration of theory-based practice has begun at Cedars as a result of the conferences. A committee composed of nursing unit directors, supervisors, clinical specialists, and educators has been formed to study nursing theories that could be practiced on individual units or hospital-wide. Savina Schoenhofer, associate professor and Graduate Program Director at Florida Atlantic University, is working with us as we explore theoretical frameworks. Nursing units involved in theory-based practice will choose, test, and evaluate specific nursing theories. I have come to know that colleagues must participate in the definition, design, and implementation of plans. Plans only succeed when they are based on the values of the profession, the staff nurses, the administration, and the institution.

Education is the vehicle to move nursing into the 21st century as a profession. Throughout my nursing career, my role as a facilitator has been very fulfilling, and I'm gratified to see the seeds planted during my journey are coming to fruition. I believe that when the creative possibilities of theory-based practice are widely known, every nurse will come along.

It has been a long journey from my original exposure to the theories of Henderson, Orem, and Peplau to the array of theories presented at the Nursing Theorist Conferences. The presentation of the practical application of these theories has been very meaningful to nurses in the south Florida community. In the last two years we have met with, been excited, enriched, and challenged by Rogers, Parse, Orem, King, Johnson, Levine, Neuman, Newman, and Watson. To me, this is a dream come true, but it is only the beginning. Practice based on theory will, in time, become the standard, ultimately benefiting the patient and increasing the professionalism of nurses.

Part 2

Johnson's Behavioral System Model for Nursing

4

The Behavioral System Model for Nursing

Dorothy E. Johnson

The behavioral system model for nursing has been in the process of development for nearly the entire course of my professional life. As a student of nursing, I was convinced that nursing had something unique and significant to offer patients—something that differs from but is complementary to the contribution made by medicine or other health professions. I was taught, and came to believe, that nursing is a profession, or at least an emerging one. This belief caused no problems for me until I began to teach in the early 1940s. I was then faced squarely with the question: what content is properly included in a course in nursing because it constitutes nursing knowledge? I found I could not differentiate nursing knowledge from medical knowledge, nor from basic science knowledge on any rational basis. This led me to still other questions: knowledge for what purpose, to what end? If nursing is a profession, then like other health professions, there is an explicit, ideal goal in patient care that only nurses are responsible for helping patients to achieve. What is this goal for nursing? The lack of answers to these questions puzzled, intrigued, and challenged me. I set myself the dual task of clarifying, at least for myself, nursing's mission and of identifying the nature of the body of knowledge necessary to reach the goal specified.

My approach to this task was threefold. In the beginning the historical approach heavily influenced me, in particular the reading of Florence Nightingale's *Notes on Nursing: What it is and what it is not*. From Nightingale, I accepted as nursing's traditional concern a focus on the person rather than the disease. The empirical approach to nursing, that is, nursing is what nurses do, came next; this was a very prominent approach in the late 1940s and early 1950s. Task studies were going on everywhere, but the tasks were so innumerable, the reasons behind them so varied, and their consequences so diverse, that the results of the studies were not only inconclusive but discouraging. This approach did help me to keep focused not just on people in general, but on people who are ill or who might be prevented from becoming ill. The third approach, an analytical one—asking what reason suggests—was the most useful one, albeit the last one used. Here I came eventually, through several progressive stages (some of which are recorded in the literature) to conceive of nursing's specific contribution to patient welfare as that of fostering efficient and effective behavioral functioning in the person both to prevent illness and during and following illness. This means a person (1) who is able to behave in a manner commensurate with social demands; (2) who is able to modify his or her behavior in ways that support biological imperatives; (3) who is able to benefit to the fullest extent during illness from the knowledge and skill of members of the health occupations; and (4) who behaves in a way that does not give evidence of unnecessary trauma as a consequence of illness.

With this focus on efficient and effective behavioral functioning, it became useful to accept a theoretical view of nursing's client, the person, as a behavioral system in much the same way that physicians have accepted a theoretical view of the person as a biological system. The acceptance of the behavioral system as the client is the primary component of this nursing model. Acceptance of this point of view is made possible by the development and rapid expansion in the last 40 years of literature contributing to our understanding of the person as a behavioral system. This interdisciplinary literature has been developed by behavioral scientists, animal and human ethnologists, biological scientists, and nursing scientists. The focus of these scientists is on the behavior of the individual as a whole—on what he or she does, why, and the consequences achieved—not on why or how the individual has changed over time in an intraorganismic sense. It is the study of the *output* of the intraorganismic structures and processes as they are coordinated and articulated, and as they respond to changes in sensory stimulation. More specifically, the focus is on social behavior—the observable features and actions of the person that take into account the actual or implied presence of other social beings. In particular the focus is on those forms of behavior that have been shown to have major adaptive significance.

An empirical literature supporting the conception of a behavioral system composed of *all* of the person's patterned and purposeful behavior is largely to be developed. There has been considerable research and theoretical attention, however, directed toward specific response systems within what I consider to be the total complex of the whole behavioral system. This is not unlike the case of knowledge about the biological system where knowledge of parts, the subsystems, preceded knowledge of the whole. Fortunately, we can tentatively rely on a developing body of knowledge about systems in general and the laws that govern the operation of all systems until further knowledge of the behavioral system as a whole is developed.

In essence, the idea behind the behavioral system model is that all the patterned, repetitive, purposeful ways of behaving that characterize each person's life make up an organized and integrated whole—a system. This system determines and limits the interactions between the person and his or her environment, and establishes the relationship of the person to the objects, events, and situations in the environment. Such behavior is orderly and predictable. It is maintained because it has been functionally efficient and effective most of the time in managing the individual's relationship to the environment. It changes when this is no longer the case, or when some more optimal level of functioning is perceived as desirable by the individual.

The behavioral system has many tasks or missions to perform in maintaining its own integrity and in managing the system's relationship to its environment. The parts of the system evolve, or the subsystems develop, each to carry out its own specialized tasks for the system as a whole. Each subsystem is composed of a set of behavioral responses, or responsive tendencies or action systems, that seem to share a common drive or goal. Organized around drives (or some type of intraorganismic motivational structure), these responses are differentiated, developed, and modified through maturation, experience, and learning. They are determined and are continuously governed by a multitude of physical, biological, psychological, and social factors operating in a complex and interlocking fashion. These behavioral action systems can be readily observed.

Consider, for example, the proximity-seeking or contact-seeking behavior so clearly seen in infants and young children. The visual seeking and following by the infant of the caretaker is an early form of attachment behavior that progresses with growth to such actions as turning, creeping toward, following on foot, reaching for, holding onto, and hugging the caretaker. Under usual conditions, these behaviors stimulate the caretaker's reinforcing responses of contact, regarding, smiling, talking to, picking up, and so forth. Such attachment behavior is modified over time and may become so subtle in adults as to be difficult to discern, but it is there except for aberrant cases. The telephone company advertisement that reminds us to "reach out and touch someone" is a valid indicator of the importance of attachment behavior throughout life.

The subsystems are linked and open, and a disturbance in one is likely to have an effect on others. Although each has a specialized task, the system as a whole depends upon an integrated performance. The subsystems now identified are seven: affiliative or attachment, ingestive, eliminative, dependency, aggressive, sexual, and achievement. Behavioral patterns in these areas are found cross-culturally and for the most part across a broad range of the phylogenetic scale. This latter connection supports the idea that these response systems, or at least the primary releasers for them, are genetically programmed. The great variability in human responses also points to the significance of social and cultural factors in their development. The ultimate group of response systems to be included within the behavioral system may well change over time on the basis of new knowledge.

The structural components of the behavioral subsystems are incompletely known although we know there is structure inherent in every system. Only the actual behavior can be directly observed, but inferences can be made as to the native of the components of the subsystems by studying the form the behavior takes (its organization and patterning), the significant ambient variables, and the consequences achieved by the behavior. The first, and perhaps most significant of the components is the *drive*—that which is a stimulant to action; or if looked at from the other direction, the *goal*—that which is sought. Another component that has substantial empirical support is the *set*, or predisposition to act (with reference to the goal) in certain ways rather than other ways. The third component is formed by the totality of the behavioral repertoire available to the individual for the achievement of a particular goal—the individual's *choices*. The fourth component is made up of the *actions*—the organized and patterned behavior directly observed. Further research is needed to verify and/or modify our knowledge of the structural components of the subsystems, as well as our understanding of the structure of the behavioral system as a whole.

The brief discussion of the identified response systems and their functions that follows is my original conception and the one to which I still subscribe. This point needs to be emphasized since major changes to the model have been made over the years by those using it, and these changes have appeared in the literature. The changes are such that they alter the fundamental nature of the behavioral system as originally proposed, and I do not agree with them.

One of the first response systems to emerge developmentally is the attachment or affiliative subsystem. It is probably the most critical subsystem for it forms the basis for all social organization. At its most general level it serves the function of security (survival), while more empirically it has the consequence of social inclusion, intimacy, and formation of social bonds. The literature on attachment behavior, particularly in the infant and young child is a rich and growing one.

Descriptions and explanations of dependency behavior have been found in the literature for a long time, but this response system served as a kind of umbrella concept that included attachment. With the separating out of attachment behavior and its functions, dependency behavior appears to have more limited and precise functions. In the broadest sense it is succoring behavior that calls for a response of nurturance. More specifically, it is behavior that seeks approval, attention, recognition, and physical assistance. Developmentally, dependency behavior in the socially optimum case evolves from almost total dependence on others to a greater degree of dependence on self, with a certain amount of interdependence essential to the survival of social groups.

Because of the association of the ingestive and eliminative subsystems with the biological system, it is important to make clear that these response systems, as parts of the behavior system, have to do with when, how, what, how much, and under what conditions we eat and when, how, and under what conditions we eliminate. Ingestive behavior can thus be seen to serve the broad function of appetitive satisfaction in its own right. This may be and all too often is at odds with biological requirements for goods and fluids. When, how, how much, and under what conditions we eat are all governed by biological, social, and psychological considerations far more potent than food itself even among the poor and hungry. The function of the eliminative subsystem is more difficult to differentiate from that of the biological system, yet clearly all humans (and many animals) must learn expected modes of behavior in the excretion of wastes, and these behaviors often take precedence over or strongly influence otherwise purely biological acts.

The sexual subsystem also has strong biological underpinnings, though we are more likely to recognize that biological factors play only one role in the sexual behavior expected and learned in any given culture. With its dual functions of procreation and gratification, this response system probably originates with the development of a gender role identity and covers the broad range of those behaviors dependent upon that identity, including but not limited to courting and mating.

The postulated function of the aggressive subsystem is self (and societal) protection and preservation. This follows the thinking of animal behaviorists rather than that of the behavioral reinforcement school which maintains that aggressive behavior is not only learned, but has as its primary intent the injury of others. It should be noted, however, that even in animal societies, the imperatives of collective life demand that limits be placed on self-protective behavior and that there must be protection and respect for life and property.

Development of the achievement subsystem probably is first manifested by exploratory behavior and attempts to manipulate the environment. Its function is mastery or control of some aspect of self or environment as measured against some standard of excellence. The significance of intellectual achievement behavior has long been recognized, but there are other areas in which achievement behavior also has been described; these are physical, creative, mechanical, and social skills. Still other areas may emerge with further research; tentatively included now are care-taking skills, which include care of children, spouses, and home.

With this conception of the patient as a behavioral system, the primary goal in patient care is thought to be behavioral system balance and dynamic stability. The need for nursing arises when there are disturbances in the structure or function of the system as a whole or in one or more subsystems, or when behavioral functioning is at a less than desired level for the individual. Nursing is seen as an external regulatory force that acts to preserve the organization and integration of the patient's behavior at the highest possible level under those conditions in which the behavior constitutes a threat to physical or social health, or in which illness is found. This force operates through the temporary imposition of external regulatory or control mechanisms in attempt to fulfill the functional requirements of the subsystems or change their structural components in desirable ways.

More specifically, the nursing diagnostic and treatment process requires first the determination of the existence of a problem. Through interview, a family and individual behavioral system history, past and present, is acquired. Structured and unstructured observation, together with other objective methodologies, are used to verify and expand that information. Investigation is directed toward the organization of the behavioral system as a whole, and two major questions are considered. First, is the patient's behavior efficient and effective in obtaining the outcomes he or she seeks? Subsidiary questions focus on the amount of energy being used to achieve desired goals, the compatibility of the behavior with survival imperatives or its congruence with the social situation, and the person's degree of satisfaction with his or her behavior. The second major question is whether the behavior is orderly, purposeful, and predictable. If the answer to either of these two major questions is no, further investigation is needed.

Attention is then directed toward each of the subsystems and their structural components. One needs detailed information about the drive, set, choices, and actions—for example, the drive strength, direction, and value to the individual; the solidity and specificity of the set; the range of behavior patterns available to the individual; and the usual behavior of the individual under given conditions and its effectiveness in goal attainment. Next, information is required about the organization, interaction, and integration of the subsystems; for example, is there a hierarchy of the subsystems or are any of the subsystems in conflict. On the basis of the study of this information, one or more impressions can be reached as to the nature of the problems.

Some tentative suggestions have been made about a diagnostic classification scheme that I will not attempt to go into in detail at this time. Suffice it to say three classes of internal subsystem problems have been postulated. First, there are those that arise because the functional requirements of the subsystems are not being met; that is, the subsystems are not getting adequate nourishment, stimulation, or protection. Second, there are the problems that result from some inconsistency or disharmony among the structural components of the subsystems. Third, problems occur when the behavior is disapproved or punished by the ambient culture; that is, behavior appropriate in one setting becomes culturally unacceptable in another. There are also at least two classes of intersystem problems: first, problems that arise because one (or perhaps two) subsystems dominate the entire system and second, problems that arise as a result of a conflict between two or more subsystems.

Knowledge about how systems in general operate and of the structure and function of the behavioral subsystems points the way toward the means of managing the nursing problems identified. If the functional requirements of one or more of the subsystems have not been met, then the nurse must provide the conditions and resources essential for meeting these requirements; nursing actions here may include information giving, role modeling, attention to the food being offered or the way in which it is being served, and seeing that infants or young children have access to their parents or elderly people to their pets. If there is a failure in the behavioral system's regulatory or control mechanisms, then the nurse may impose, temporarily, external controls to inhibit, stimulate, or reinforce certain behaviors. The third general approach to management of behavioral system problems is to attempt to repair disordered structural components; this is the most difficult approach since it involves changes in the drive (goal), the set, the choices, and the behavior itself and requires such things as attitudinal changes, redirection of goals, and sometimes reduction in drive strength. Management of these kinds of problems is likely to improve through our experience and increased knowledge.

One criticism of the behavioral system model has been that it does not allow for or focus attention on prevention—but that is not true. The fact is, however, that like medicine where problems in the biological system cannot be prevented until the nature of the problem is fully explained, preventive nursing is not possible until problems in the behavioral system are explicated. To the extent that any problem that might arise can be anticipated, and appropriate methodologies are available, preventive action is in order.

In summary, the behavioral system model for nursing practice is based upon substantial and steadily increasing scientific knowledge. It provides one way of conceptualizing the people nursing serves and is commensurate with what nurses and the public perceive as nursing's function. It provides a rational orientation to practice, a basis for organizing curricula, and a clear direction for research. Research in nursing practice, based on this model, is in its infancy, but there is a slowly growing number of reports of investigations and the future for theory development seems bright.

To use this model effectively in practice, intensive study of the rich literature available on the seven response systems is essential. The nurse must know, for example, how these systems develop over time, the many factors that influence that development, the cultural variations in the basic response systems to be expected, and much more. The nurse must also acquire an understanding of how living systems operate. Only with such knowledge and understanding is it possible for the practitioner to be aware of the kinds of data needed about the individual. Only with such knowledge can the practitioner analyze that data and intervene effectively.

To openly use a nursing model is risk-taking behavior for the individual nurse. For a nursing department to adopt one of these models for unit or institution use is risk-taking behavior of an even higher order. The reward for such risk-taking for the individual practitioner lies in the great satisfaction gained from being able to specify explicit concrete *nursing* goals in the care of patients and from documenting the actual achievement of the desired outcomes. The reward for the nursing department is having a rational, cohesive, and comprehensive basis for the development of standards of nursing practice, for the evaluation of practitioners, and for the documentation of the contribution of nursing to patient welfare. As more and more nurses and institutions use a specific nursing model as a basis for nursing practice, and as the outcomes of that practice are documented, evidence will accumulate as to the relative value of each model used. The ultimate social tests of the significance of nursing decisions and actions in the lives of patients; the congruence (and acceptability) of these actions with social expectations; and the utility of any particular model for nursing education, practice, and research will be satisfied. Only in this manner will nursing's social mission and our special realm of original responsibility in patient care be fully clarified.

REFERENCE

Johnson, D. E. (1980). The behavioral system model of nursing. In J. Riehl and C. Roy (Eds.). *Conceptual Models for Nursing Practice* (2nd ed.), (pp. 207–216). New York: Appleton-Century-Crofts.

5

Implementation of the Johnson Model: One Hospital's Experience

Vivien Dee

A decade of work devoted to the application of the Johnson Behavioral System Model at the UCLA Neuropsychiatric Institute and Hospital (NPH) provides an example of how a conceptual model of nursing is translated into practice. As Dorothy Johnson said, "To openly use a nursing model is risk-taking behavior for the individual nurse; for a nursing department to adopt one of these models for unit or institution use is risk-taking behavior of an even higher order." This paper will present some of the practical issues that have arisen in the course of implementing the Johnson Behavioral System Model at NPH and will provide an update on Johnson Model applications for the 1990s.

KEY POINTS TO CONSIDER

There are two key points to consider prior to the implementation of a nursing model within an institution, namely: who should decide on the selection of a nursing theory and should one or more theories be chosen?

Who Should Decide on the Selection of a Nursing Theory?

Barbara Stevens (1979), in *Nursing Theory: Analysis, Application, Evaluation* poses several questions. Should the administrative structure of an institution favor one nursing theory over another? Should the administration be eclectic, allowing each practitioner to select and implement the theory of his or her choice? Should nursing administration perceive theory selection as a right of the individual practitioner and purposely stay out of the theory business altogether? Stevens concluded that nursing administration has the ultimate responsibility for determining the structure within which care will be delivered and part of this responsibility is selecting the theoretical framework, if one is desired, within which that care will be structured. There are several reasons for this view. First, it would be costly for each unit of the institution to develop the necessary materials to support differing models of nursing. Second, the use of varying models by practitioners in the same setting would severely limit continuity of care and could result in conflicting interventions and problem identification. Whether an institution organizes care on a primary model or team model, nursing requires multiple caregivers to account for the provision of services 24 hours a day, seven days a week. It is important, therefore, that all caregivers have a common frame of reference concerning those patient factors considered to be significant for assessment as well as proposed interventions. A unified model of nursing provides just such a common frame of reference. The decision to use and select a nursing theory to guide nursing practice at NPH was an administrative one. It was this author's belief and commitment that the use of a nursing theory would guide the practice of nurses, enhance the professional base of nursing, and improve the quality of nursing care at NPH (Auger & Dee, 1982).

Should One or More Theories Be Chosen?

This question requires both managerial as well as theoretical considerations. The reasons in support for a single unified theory have already been presented, namely: (1) its cost effectiveness in relation to such things as the development of forms, teaching materials, and procedures and (2) the need for a common frame of reference for all staff. A single theory implemented institution-wide facilitates the coordination and continuity of care for patients who may be transferred from one unit to another. The education of nursing staff is also facilitated when a single theory is selected. Additionally, a single theory approach enables the nurse executive to interpret more effectively the domains of nursing practice to physicians and administrators. At NPH, the single theory approach is used.

SELECTION OF A THEORY

The Johnson Behavioral System Model was selected for three major reasons. First, the model focuses on observable behaviors of the patient with which nursing is concerned, thereby delineating nursing's distinct contribution to patient care. Second, the model identifies universal patterns of behavior applicable to all individuals regardless of age, cultural differences, or medical diagnosis. Finally, the model emphasizes the bio-psycho-social and cultural factors influencing behavior, thereby permitting the model's application in all clinical settings.

SETTING

NPH is a 209-bed tertiary care and major teaching medical center of the University of California at Los Angeles. The Johnson Model is implemented in the child and adult psychiatric inpatient services. The child service includes a child and an adolescent psychiatry unit, and a child and an adolescent developmental disabilities unit. The adult service includes two general adult psychiatry units and a geropsychiatry unit. Patients admitted to the inpatient units range from age two to over 90. Average length of stay in the childrens' service is 49 days while average length of stay in the adult service is 19 days.

IMPLEMENTATION

Auger & Dee (1983) began their work in 1978 with the formulation of a general framework operationalizing the Johnson Model for direct applicability to the clinical setting of psychiatry. Each behavioral subsystem was operationalized in terms of its specific definitions and behavioral characteristics. The amplified version of the Johnson Model, which included Johnson's seven subsystems plus the restorative subsystem described by Auger (1976), provided the original theoretical framework for the development of the NPH Patient Classification Instrument (PCI). The PCI was designed to have both clinical and administrative applications; consequently, it is composed of two parts. The first part lists behaviors representing varying degrees of adaptiveness to maladaptiveness. These behavioral indices serve as the basis for the clinical assessment of patient behaviors. The second part lists nursing interventions based on the level of care the patient requires, from minimal care to continuous one-to-one care—thereby permitting the determination of workload on the basis of patient care needs.

Prior to implementing the Johnson Model on the four child and adolescent inpatient units in April 1981, it was necessary to revise existing nursing assessment forms, develop teaching materials, conduct seminars for the orientation of staff to the model, and design a general orientation class for new employees. To facilitate staff learning, an interview guide was developed to assist nurses in eliciting information from the patient and family. The interview guide not only emphasized the assessment of critical patient behaviors, but also the assessment of the regulatory factors such as developmental, bio-physical, sociocultural, psychological, and family that may affect patients' behaviors. Following an extensive program of orientation, the nursing assessment and care plans of all newly admitted patients were based on the Johnson Model (Dee & Auger, 1983).

Once all staff had been oriented to the clinical and administrative components of the PCI, the shift coordinators (team leaders) on the child and adolescent inpatient units began to report the levels of nursing care requirements for all patients on the unit at the end of each shift. This data provided the basis for the determination of staffing on each unit according to preliminary estimates of the nursing care hours required for each level of nursing care.

Although clinical implementation of the Johnson Model did not occur on the three adult psychiatry and geropsychiatry inpatient units until 1987, administrative implementation occurred in 1982 with the shift coordinators reporting required levels of care on the basis of preliminary estimates for determining staffing. To facilitate the process of implementation on the adult service, existing Johnson Model-based assessment forms were revised to include demographic data pertinent not only for the planning of care for the child and adolescent patients, but also for the adult and geriatric patients.

By 1988, preliminary estimates for determining staffing needs were replaced with established nursing care hour parameters for each level of nursing care according to the categories of patient behaviors on each of the seven inpatient units. These established parameters, derived from a two-year observational study (Dee, 1986), are used by shift coordinators and nurse managers to calculate staffing resource needs on both the child and adult services.

As expected, the introduction of the Johnson Model into the practice setting was not met entirely with open arms and gratitude. The problem of resistance to change of any sort is ever present. There will always be staff who are going to resist new approaches, and depending on their level of influence in the work setting, their resistance can make or break the change. However, once the classes were given and the model implemented, staff resistance and objections decreased. Many staff members have commented that the availability of the framework helps them organize their thoughts and observations of patient behavior and provides a way to monitor patient progress throughout hospitalization.

The process of implementing a nursing model institution-wide has required ongoing orientation and inservice education for all staff. New nurses entering the institution require orientation and supervision on the application of a theoretical framework, while the more experienced and skillful nurses require advanced clinical seminars for ongoing dialogue on the refinement of theoretical concepts.

CURRENT DEVELOPMENTS

The current formulation of the general framework operationalizing the Johnson Model represents a return to much of Johnson's original conceptualization, including modifications of Auger's interpretations as well as amplifications by Dee & Randell (1989) on Johnson's metaparadigm concepts of person, health, nursing, and environment.

Person is represented by subsystem behaviors. Appendix 5-1 presents the revised interpretations of the eight subsystems and their associated behaviors. Health is denoted by system balance, and nursing actions are those that preserve the organization and integration of the patient's behavior by fulfilling the functional requirements of the subsystems through nurturance, protection, and stimulation. The revised version of the PCI is presented in table 5-1. Appendix 5-2 presents a sample of the formulation of Category 2 affiliative subsystem behavioral indices and nursing interventions for Level 2 nursing care on the basis of the general framework in table 5-1. Environment is represented by regulatory factors that affect subsystem behaviors. The environmental regulators are defined in appendix 5-3. Ongoing clinical projects include: (1) developing Johnson Model-based standardized care plans; (2) formulating nursing diagnoses that nurses, by virtue of their education and experience, are capable and licensed to treat; and (3) determining the criteria for evaluating patient outcomes. To date, 36 Johnson Model-based standardized nursing care plans have been completed. Appendix 5-4 presents a partial list of standardized nursing care plans by nursing diagnoses. Portions of a sample standardized care plan developed for the Child Inpatient Unit are shown in figure 5-1.

CONCLUSION

The benefits of using a nursing model in the practice setting are many. The Johnson Model (1) provides a comprehensive and systematic method of assessing patient behaviors, (2) facilitates the identification of specific areas of patient strengths and weaknesses

Table 5-1
Criteria for Rating Patient Behavior Category and Level of Nursing Interventions Required

Patient Behaviors		Nursing Interventions
CATEGORY 1 Patient demonstrates behaviors/actions that are effective and compatible in all eight subsystems, therefore achieving system balance. Energy may be unequally distributed among the eight subsystems but not to the detriment of any one subsystem or to the system as a whole. **System balance denotes health.**	I	**LEVEL 1** Category 1 patients demonstrate system balance; therefore they are able to protect, nurture and stimulate all behavioral subsystems. **The patient requires a minimum amount of nursing time in supervision and nursing care.** The primary goal of nursing care for the Category 1 patient is the provision of a nurturing and stimulating environment within a group context.
CATEGORY 2 Patient demonstrates behaviors/actions that are inconsistently effective in one or more subsystems resulting in short-term incompatibility among the subsystems and the potential for system imbalance. Energy may be temporarily distributed unequally among the subsystems creating ineffective subsystem functioning but not to the detriment of the system as a whole. **Potential for system imbalance results in the potential for health deviation.**	II	**LEVEL 2** Category 2 patients demonstrate a potential for system imbalance; therefore they are not able to consistently protect, nurture and stimulate all behavioral subsystems. **The patient requires a moderate amount of nursing time in supervision and nursing care.** The primary goal of nursing care for the Category 2 patient is the provision of a nurturing, stimulating and protective environment within a group context.
CATEGORY 3 Patient demonstrates behaviors/actions that are incompatible within one or more subsystems resulting in system imbalance and incompatibility among subsystems. Energy is unequally distributed among the eight subsystems and frequently results in the detriment of the system as a whole. **System imbalance results in illness.**	III	**LEVEL 3** Category 3 patients demonstrate system imbalance; therefore they are not able to protect, nurture and stimulate all behavioral subsystems. **The patient requires an intensive amount of nursing time in supervision and nursing care.** The primary goal of nursing care for the Category 3 patient is the provision of a nurturing and protective environment on an individual level or within a small group.
CATEGORY 4 Patient demonstrates behaviors/actions that are highly incompatible within one or more subsystems resulting in system imbalance and severe incompatibility among the subsystems that threatens survival. Energy is unequally distributed among the subsystems and this distribution of energy is of such acute intensity, long duration and/or high frequency that detriment to the system as a whole is evident. **Severe system imbalance results in critical illness.**	IV	**LEVEL 4** Category 4 patients demonstrate severe system imbalance; therefore they are not able to protect, nurture and stimulate all behavioral subsystems. **The patient requires continuous one-to-one supervision and nursing care.** The primary goal of nursing care for the Category 4 patient is the provision of a nurturing and protective environment on an individual level.

Source: UCLA Neuropsychiatric Institute and Hospital

Figure 5-1
Portions of a Standardized Care Plan

ADDRESSOGRAPH

UCLA NEUROPSYCHIATRIC HOSPITAL
PSYCHIATRIC INPATIENT SERVICES
NURSING SERVICES
TREATMENT PLAN
(A Component of the Psychiatric Inpatient Services Multi-disciplinary Treatment Plan)

NURSING DIAGNOSIS SUBSYSTEM CODES:
1. Ingestive   5. Affiliative
2. Eliminative   6. Aggressive-Protective
3. Dependency   7. Sexual
4. Achievement   8. Restorative

MASTER PROBLEM:

DATE AND SIGNATURE	EVIDENCED BY:	NURSING DIAGNOSIS Note: one diagnosis/problem per page

	Poor Social Skills:
	☐ teasing
	☐ provocative behavior
	☐ name calling
	☐ stealing
	☐ verbal conflicts with peers
	☐ interrupts others' conversations
	☐ lack of awareness of personal space
	☐ other (specify)
	
	Negative Attention Seeking:
	☐ oppositional
	☐ noncompliant
	☐ argumentative
	☐ tantrums
	☐ fabrication
	☐ other (specify)
		☐ Insufficiency of the ____ Subsystem
		☐ Discrepancy of the ____ Subsystem
		☐ Dominance of the ____ Subsystem over the ____ Subsystem
		☒ Incompatibility between the _3_ Subsystem and the _5_ Subsystem
		
		RELATED TO: ☐ Bio-physical ☒ Psychological ☒ Family
		☐ Developmental ☐ Sociocultural ☐ Physical Environmental
		
		Psychological - Attention Deficit Disorder with Hyperactivity.
		Family - Parents divorced one year ago, lives with mother, sees father infrequently, mother is clinically depressed and states she cannot manage child's behavior.
		
		DISCHARGE OUTCOMES/LONG TERM GOALS: By discharge, the patient will participate in all activities/programs using appropriate social skills without evidence of negative attention-seeking.
		
		NURSING INTERVENTION
		1. To teach/facilitate effective social interactions and decrease ineffective affiliative and attention-seeking behaviors, assigned staff will:
		   ☐ a. Encourage patient to initiate social interactions with peers
		   ☐ b. Role model conversational behavior (i.e., topics, appropriate assertion, moderate voice volume, asking for help and/or attention).
			PREDICTED OUTCOME/SHORT TERM GOALS
			(include time Frame)
			
			☐ By ____, patient will meet with staff ____ times per shift for sessions and feedback.
			
			☐ By ____, patient will verbally state one effective social behavior to use in interactions with peers.

Source: UCLA Neuropsychiatric Institute and Hospital

in ways that are observable and measurable, (3) enhances consistency and continuity of care, (4) promotes the organization of diverse data into meaningful segments, (5) prioritizes the provision of care on the basis of an understanding of subsystem interactions, (6) promotes a common language and unity in the practice environment, (7) facilitates a sense of professional identity, and (8) enhances the equitable allocation of resources according to variable patient care needs rather than the allocation of resources merely by census.

The Johnson Model has provided nurses with a framework not only to describe phenomena, but also to explain, predict, and control clinical phenomena for the purpose of achieving desired patient outcomes. Levels of nursing care provided for the patient are, therefore, purposeful and nursing practice is more meaningful for the practitioner.

The challenge to nurse executives is to create environments that promote optimal professional practice so that the quality of patient care can be sustained and further enhanced.

Appendix 5-1
Subsystems and Associated Behaviors

1. Ingestive: Behavior associated with food and fluid intake.
2. Eliminative: Behavior associated with patterns of elimination.
3. Dependency: Behavior associated with methods of seeking approval, attention, and recognition.
4. Affiliative: Behavior associated with patterns of relating.
5. Aggressive-Protective: Behavior associated with the protection of self from perceived and/or real harm.
6. Sexual: Behavior associated with gender, intimacy, and procreation.
7. Achievement: Behavior associated with mastery of self-help, independent living, problem-solving, and decision making.
8. Restorative: Behavior associated with sleep and rest.

Appendix 5-2
Example of Level 2 Nursing Interventions for Treatment of Category 2 Behaviors Related to Patient's Affiliative Subsystem

Patient Behavior Indices	Nursing Interventions
• Demonstrates difficulty in forming emotional attachments to significant others.	• Provide specific time for establishing relationships with staff and peers.
• Establishes and/or maintains limited relationships with peers and/or others.	• Maintain treatment plan to facilitate group participation.
• Relates in superficial or inappropriate manner.	• Provide periodic prompts/reinforcements for effective communication.
• Establishes and maintains limited relationships in group settings and activities.	• Maintain treatment plan to facilitate interactions with family and significant others.
• Demonstrates difficulty in communicating ideas and feelings in verbal, non-verbal, and written forms.	• Provide periodic verbal/physical reinforcement to assist establishment of social/physical boundaries.
• Initiates and maintains communication infrequently and/or ineffectively.	• Clarify interactions with others.
• Demonstrates difficulty maintaining social and physical boundaries as distinct from those of other people.	• Provide periodic orientation to staff, daily activities, and unit routine.

Appendix 5-3
Definitions of Environmental Regulators

Internal Regulators
Bio-physical: Physiological status, medical condition or diagnosis, medication, and treatments.
Psychological: Self-perception, cognitive functioning, and coping styles.
Developmental: Milestones, current level of functioning, and departures from normal progressions.

External Regulators
Sociocultural: Values, religious beliefs, economic status, ethnicity, and support systems.
Family: Structure, function, and dynamics.
Physical Environment: Home, neighborhood, and surroundings.

Appendix 5-4
Partial List of Standard Care Plans by Nursing Diagnoses

1. Insufficiency of the ingestive subsystem evidenced by failure to ingest adequate food and fluid resulting in continued severe weight loss and dehydration.
2. Incompatibility between the ingestive subsystem and the elimination subsystem evidenced by a "binge-purge" cycle.
3. Incompatibility between the dependency subsystem and the affiliative subsystem evidenced by poor social skills and negative attention seeking.
4. Insufficiency of the aggressive-protective subsystem evidenced by suicidal behavior.
5. Discrepancy of the aggressive-protective subsystem evidenced by lack of self-protection.
6. Discrepancy of the eliminative subsystem evidenced by urinary frequency, complaints of discomfort.
7. Insufficiency of the achievement subsystem evidenced by the inability to perform activities of daily living independently.
8. Insufficiency of the affiliative subsystem evidenced by isolative and/or withdrawn behavior.
9. Insufficiency of the restorative subsystem evidenced by difficulty sleeping, falling asleep, and intermittent awakening.

REFERENCES

Auger, J. (1976). *Behavioral systems and nursing.* Englewood Cliffs, NJ: Prentice-Hall, Inc.

Auger, J., & Dee, V. (1982, November). *Can a model of nursing be translated into practice?* Paper presented at the National Research Conference, Palo Alto, CA.

Auger, J., & Dee, V. (1983). A patient classification system based on the behavioral system model of nursing, Part 1. *The Journal of Nursing Administration, 13*(4), 38–43.

Dee, V., & Auger, J. (1983). A patient classification system based on the behavioral system model of nursing, Part 2. *The Journal of Nursing Administration, 13*(5), 18–23.

Dee, V. (1986). *Validation of a patient classification instrument for pyschiatric patients based on the Johnson Model of Nursing.* Dissertation Abstracts International, 47, 4822B. University of California, San Francisco, CA.

Dee, V., & Randell, B. (1989). *NPH patient classification system: A theory-based nursing practice model for staffing.* Paper presented at UCLA Neuropsychiatric Institute and Hospital, Los Angeles, CA.

Stevens, B. (1979). Nursing theory: *Analysis, application, evaluation.* Boston: Little, Brown and Company.

Part 3

Orem's Self-Care Deficit Theory of Nursing

6

A Nursing Practice Theory in Three Parts, 1956–1989

Dorothea E. Orem

Nurses and other health workers are in a new age of health care that can be for nursing a period of continuing development or a period of decline. Nurses have made nursing what it is—a service that is needed and sought by individuals and families when certain life situations prevail. Experienced nurses recognize such life situations when they encounter them and know when their work of nursing others, caring for others, or helping them care for themselves is producing beneficial results. These same nurses, however, want to be able to tell people what they do and why they do it; they want to know why their practice of nursing is effective.

The nurses who ask such questions are thinking nurses. They have vast knowledge gained from nursing practice situations. They also have knowledge of the human sciences and the medical sciences, but they do not have speculative or theoretical knowledge of nursing. Their nursing education has not made available to them the practical and applied nursing sciences. Speculative knowledge of nursing, and its use by nurses to make their practice of nursing more complete and effective, is the focus of this conference. In the absence of developed nursing sciences, nurses are taking a first step toward developing them by focusing on nursing theories that will explicate a wide range of nursing practice situations. A general theory of nursing is one that applies to all situations of practice and explains when and why nursing is needed by individuals or families, what is involved in nursing, and what results can be achieved through nursing. My task is to acquaint you with one particular general theory of nursing known as the self-care deficit nursing theory. This theory and its composing elements are expressed in the form of generalizations about persons who need, and persons who produce nursing, and about events and processes within nursing practice situations. This speculative or theoretical knowledge about nursing practice situations was formulated, expressed, and formalized through my efforts and those of my colleagues—first to understand and then to describe and continue to investigate the recurring person and process features of nursing practice situations.

Susan Taylor's task in the next chapter is to acquaint you with how nurses have used, and should use, the self-care deficit theory of nursing to guide their practice, direct their observations, and attach meaning to the concrete features of nursing practice situations. Taylor's presentation will focus on the conditions and circumstances of nursing practice situations.

FEATURES OF NURSING PRACTICE SITUATIONS

Nursing is a particular form of health care that is distinguished by certain professional, technological features. Because nursing is available in communities to some, if not to all persons who need it, nursing also has socioeconomic features. These socioeconomic features determine how nursing as a health service fits into the life of a community, how nurses come in contact with and enter into agreements with persons who need nursing, what nursing costs, and how it is paid for. Since nurses are in contact with persons for whom they provide nursing and with associates of these persons, the interpersonal features of nursing practice situations must be taken into account when nursing is described and explained. The self-care deficit theory of nursing, its broad conceptual elements, and their developed substantive elements identify, describe, and explain the professional, technological features of nursing and the related interpersonal and social features of nursing practice.

PROFESSIONAL TECHNOLOGICAL FEATURES OF THE SELF-CARE DEFICIT THEORY OF NURSING

The self-care deficit theory of nursing is understood through the theory of self-care, the theory of self-care deficit, and the theory of nursing system. This general theory of nursing is complex because nursing, as the theory explains, is a practical endeavor that requires investigative, decision-making, and production-type activities.

This three-part theory focuses not on individuals, but on persons in relations. Each of the three theories has as its focus a specific dimension of the person: the theory of self-care focuses on the self, the I; the theory of self-care deficit focuses on you and me; and the theory of nursing system focuses on we, persons in community.

The three parts of this general theory reflect the growth and development of their formulators' understandings of nursing and their search for ways to present their insights to others. For example, the ideas and elements expressed in the three theories were initially expressed as definitions of nursing. Further investigation into the question of why people need nursing led to an understanding of the proper object of nursing as those persons who are unable in whole or in part to regulate their own functioning and development through self-care because of health derived or health related action limitations or who are unable to do this for their dependents because of the dependents' health situations. Conceptual elements were isolated, defined, developed, and related until a conceptual model could be constructed.

The basis for the modeling was my own and my colleagues' understanding of deliberate human action, or conduct, or ego-processed behavior. The terminology used to name the elements of the model and the theories and their elements has its origin in the language traditionally used to describe and explain deliberate result-seeking action of human beings.

Theories are expressed through the use of conceptual elements that point, relate, and attach meaning to facts or phenomena that the theory developers understand. Understanding is a necessary condition for conceptualization. Concepts and elements of a theory are named by theory developers. The language used to describe theory may differ from our everyday use of words.

Each of the three theories within the self-care deficit nursing theory is composed of four conceptual elements. All four of the following elements are required within each theory: the conceptualized entity, persons in space-time localizations; attributes or properties of these persons; motion or change; and effects or results, what is produced.

In the following sections of this paper, the three theories are described first by their central ideas and then in terms of the four required conceptual elements.

The Theory of Self-Care

The central idea of the theory of self-care is expressed as follows:

> Maturing or mature persons contribute to the regulation of their own functioning and development and to the prevention, control, or amelioration of disease and injury and their effects by performing within the context of their day-to-day living, learned actions directed to themselves or their environments that are known or assumed to have regulatory value with respect to human functioning and development (Winstead-Fry, 1986).

This central idea is elaborated by Orem (1985) in a series of ten propositions.

The *entity* conceptualized in the theory of self-care is: maturing or mature persons who are engaging in a self-regulatory form of action named self-care that they perform within the context of their day-to-day living. The theory of self-care assumes three conceptualized *properties* or attributes of such persons: (1) having requirements for regulation of human functioning and development (self-care requisites) that can be met only through the deliberate selection and performance of appropriate care measures,

(2) having the ability to manage self within a stable or changing environment, and (3) having developing or developed capabilities to identify and particularize regulatory requirements and being able to meet those requirements through the timed use of known valid and reliable care measures or through trial and error. The complex of capabilities expressed by the third property is named the self-care agency.

Conceptualizations of *motion or change* in the self-care theory relate to both persons engaged in self-care and to their properties or attributes. In terms of persons who engage in self-care, motion is conceptualized in terms of change from one kind of self-care operation to another, or from not being engaged in self-care to being engaged in self-care operations in some sequence of performance. The forms of self-care operations are identified as investigative operations, transitional or decision-making operations, and productive operations (the ones through which regulation of human functioning and development is effected).

Change in the properties of persons who engage in self-care is also a part of the theory of self-care. Change in regulatory requirements or self-care requisites within the theory of self-care is understood in relation to three types of requisites: universal, developmental, and health deviation. The particularized values of universal and developmental type requisites may change as well as the ways and means for meeting them. Health deviation requisites may or may not be present and if present may change in both number and kind. Self-management capabilities may increase or decrease in quality or quantity. Self-care agency may continue to develop, may stabilize, or may decrease in value.

The *product* or result of persons' regulatory actions to control internal as well as environmental factors is conceptualized as a self-care system constituted from articulated actions that are performed in some sequence. The performed actions that constitute the self-care system determine the regulatory results that are achievable. Since self-care under ordinary internal and external conditions is performed in large part out of habit, persons' self-care systems present some enduring characteristics.

Persons who engage in the regulatory function of self-care and the three named properties of the person are subject to human and environmental factors. For example, the health state of a person affects the presence or absence of health deviation self-care requisites. It is helpful in an effort to understand the theory to relate the factors known to affect the four identified conceptual elements.

The factors that have a basic or foundational effect on the elements conceptualized in the theory of self-care are age, gender, developmental state, culture, health state, family system, health care system, environmental condition, socioeconomic situation, resources, pattern of living, and life experiences.

Through the performance of the investigative and transitional self-care operations, existent values of the active basic conditioning factors are brought into the focus and consideration of the self-care agent (the person engaged in self-care). These values are related to existent or emerging self-care requisites and ways and means for meeting them. The product of these operations is the calculated demand for engagement in self-care, known as the *therapeutic self-care demand*. The performance of the investigative and transitional self-care operations also requires the relating of the conditioning effects of human and environmental factors to self-management capabilities and to self-care agency. This relating ends in judgments about the adequacy of these capabilities in meeting some or all components of the therapeutic self-care demand. A component of a therapeutic self-care demand is constituted from a particularized self-care requisite, a selected means for meeting it, and the care measures (sets of actions) required to use the means to meet the requisite.

Theory of Self-Care Deficit

The central idea of the theory of self-care deficit expresses why individuals require and can be helped through nursing.

> The self-care agency of mature and maturing individuals in relation to their knowing and meeting their therapeutic self-care demands can be adversely affected by health-associated conditions and factors internal or external to such individuals that render their self-care agency wholly or partially non-operational or qualitatively inadequate for knowing and meeting their

therapeutic self-care demands and thus giving rise to legitimate requirements for nursing (Winstead-Fry, 1986).

This central idea is further developed by Orem (1985) in a series of six propositions.

The *entity* conceptualized in the theory of self-care deficit is defined as those persons whose self-care agency is inadequate for knowing and meeting all or some of the components of their therapeutic self-care demands. The *attributes* specified for these persons is the presence of existent or emerging limitations for performing self-care operations. Limitations for the effective performance of estimative, transitional, or productive operations or for all of these are identified within the theory as health derived or health related. For example, the health state of a person may limit either the kinds of actions persons can perform or specify the actions they should perform.

The *motion or change* conceptualized is found within persons with self-care deficits or in the persons who act for them. Included are recognition of existent or emerging self-care or dependent-care limitations, identification that nursing is a needed service, and seeking and accepting nursing.

Two *products* are conceptualized. The first is an agreement between persons with health derived or health related self-care or dependent-care deficits and nurses to take on their appropriate roles and responsibilities within a nursing practice situation. The second product is the initiation and beginning development of an interpersonal relationship that permits communication and moves toward interpersonal unity involving association, interaction, and integration, as well as recognition and acceptance of the independence and interdependence implicit in any differentiation of roles and responsibilities within the nursing situation. Interpersonal unity is characterized by an active, operative dynamic sense of duty on the part of nurses, the persons with self-care deficits (when competent), and the relatives or associates of those persons.

The factors identified in the theory of self-care as basic conditioners of persons or their properties are also important elements within the theory of self-care deficit. Age, gender, developmental state, family system, life experiences, and pattern of living are useful for describing persons with existent or potential self-care deficits. Description includes persons' general action capabilities and developmental potentials. Health state, health-care system, and developmental state are viewed as existent or potential sources of self-care action limitations and as generators of self-care requisites. Such factors also affect how and if existent self-care requisites can be met. These factors and others condition what motion or change can or does take place toward the formation of nursing practice situations and interpersonal relationships.

Theory of Nursing System

The theory of nursing system is the most complex of the three theories. Its central idea relates to the movements and products specified by the theory of self-care deficit, namely, the movement to seek and accept nursing, the agreement to provide and receive nursing, and the institution of interpersonal relationships between persons who agree to provide nursing and those who agree to participate in the service.

> All action systems that are nursing systems are produced by nurses through the exercise of nursing agency within the context of their contracted and interpersonal relations with [persons] who are characterized by health associated self-care deficits for purposes of ensuring that their therapeutic self-care demands are known and met and their self-care agency is protected or its exercise or development is regulated (Winstead-Fry, 1986).

This central idea is elaborated by Orem (1985) in a set of eight propositions.

The *entity* conceptualized in the theory of nursing system is an interpersonal unity in a particular time-space localization. This unity is formed by nurses, persons who have entered into an agreement to accept and participate in nursing, and the relatives or persons who are responsible for the individuals who require nursing. The unity is something that must be continuously maintained by communication, coordination of actions, and cooperation among the persons forming the unity. Each person within the unity ideally recognizes the independence as well as the interdependence of the individuals involved, and each person ideally brings an active, operative sense of duty to the nursing situation.

The *attributes* or *properties* conceptualized within the theory of nursing system are attributed to the interpersonal unity and to the persons who are essential to the initiation, development, and continued existence of the unity of persons that enables the nursing. Attributes are considered from both the societal perspective and the perspective of the production of nursing.

From a societal perspective the relationships specified by an agreement or contract for nursing must meet the legal requirements specified by the jurisdiction where the nursing is offered. From a nursing perspective the relationships must exhibit nursing legitimacy. This means that there is evidence of existent, emerging, or potential self-care deficit (or dependent-care deficit) on the part of the persons seeking nursing and evidence of the necessary knowledge and capabilities on the part of the providers of nursing.

The *attributes* conceptualized for persons within the unity are (1) the state of development and operability of the self-care or dependent-care agency of the persons requiring nursing and the inadequacy of their agency for knowing and meeting their existent or emerging therapeutic self-care demands, and (2) the property of nursing agency on part of nurses, that is, the capabilities necessary to perform the essential operations of nursing practice (nursing diagnosis, prescription, and regulation) for and with persons who require nursing.

The *motion or change* conceptualized refers to the unity, the persons forming it, and their properties. Communication between and among members of the unity and the time, place, conditions, and circumstances of that communication constitute motion or change and thus affect the maintenance of the unity. The unity is functional as a nursing unity when nurses activate their powers of nursing agency in order to know and meet the therapeutic self-care demands of the persons who require nursing and to regulate the exercise or development of their self-care agency. More specific changes include increases or decreases in dependence, independence, and interdependence of persons within the interpersonal unity and changes in role responsibilities.

With respect to persons and properties, persons requiring nursing may have increases or decreases in the number and kind of self-care capabilities and limitations, increase or decrease in willingness to participate in nursing, increase or decrease in the number and kinds of self-care requisites or changes in available means of meeting them, and increase or decrease in engagement in self-care or in regulation of the exercise or development of self-care agency. Persons who are nurses are conceptualized as moving from the performance of one nursing practice operation to performance of another operation, from use of one or more methods of helping to the use of one or more other methods of helping, and from willingness to maintain the nursing relationship to movement to end it.

The *products* conceptualized within the theory of nursing system include the establishment of role functions for persons within the nursing unity, the design for performance of the differentiated roles in a time-place matrix, and the emergence and maintenance of stable or changing nursing systems through performance of role functions by the persons within the nursing unity. The selection of valid and appropriate ways of helping; the allocation of role functions to nurses, persons who require nursing, and other persons involved; and the performance of those role functions determine the form of nursing systems.

The results of nursing are understood and expressed within the theory of nursing system in relation to the two patient or client variables, namely, their therapeutic self-care demands and their self-care agency. Results of nursing include (1) persons within the nursing unity having knowledge of the components of therapeutic self-care demands and the regulatory value of each component as related to human functioning and development, (2) effective meeting of components of therapeutic self-care demands in time specific sequences, (3) regulation of the exercise and development of self-care or dependent-care agency, and (4) nurses' knowledge and judgments about the need to alter the form of the nursing system, to continue it, or to move to a dependent-care or self-care system.

It is the validity and the reliability of the technologies selected to meet particularized self-care requisites as well as the accuracy of the identification and particularization of requisites that determine whether or not desirable levels of regulation of human functioning and development are achieved. Such results may or may not be immediately perceptible to members of the nursing unity. When self-care requisites exist but cannot be met because of the absence of valid or reliable technologies, when the use of technologies to meet one requisite interferes with the meeting of other requisites, when there is reluctance or refusal to use certain technologies, and/or when structural or functional conditions do not permit regulatory action, then the nursing system and the results expected from it must be adjusted to reflect the existent conditions.

The factors that are understood to condition the persons, properties, movement, and products conceptualized and related in the theory of nursing system are aspects of extrinsic systems that are linked to and interactive with the nursing system. The particular health care organizational system that accepts persons to receive nursing—for example, a clinic, hospital, or visiting nurse association, influences not only the composition of the nursing unity of interacting persons but also their time-place localizations. Health care systems are linked in a number of ways to governmental systems for the regulation and control of health care within particular jurisdictions. The governmental system conditions where nursing can be provided, how it will be financed, who will provide the service, and in some instances the quantity of service that will be provided. These systems exert extrinsic influences on the nursing system in the form of opportunities or constraints.

Other influences on nursing systems are intrinsic to the persons within the nursing unity who require nursing. The health and developmental state of persons who require nursing will affect not only nurses' selection of appropriate ways of helping and the functions to be performed, but also the extent and intensity of interactions between and among persons who constitute the nursing unity. The ages, gender, culture, and life experiences of members of the nursing unity will influence both their actions and interactions.

Major conditioners of the elements of nursing systems are other systems of health care in which persons under nursing care are concurrently participating; most commonly these are medical care systems. Medical care systems for individuals include care elements from one or more physicians utilizing some range of types of paramedical services. The way in which other systems of health care impinge upon the nursing system must be clearly understood by nurses and other members of the nursing unity.

Consider the example of Mr. X who lives as a member of the household maintained by his son and daughter-in-law. Mr. X, his daughter-in-law, and a nurse from the local visiting nurse association constitute a nursing unity formed to ensure that selected components of Mr. X's therapeutic self-care demand are known and met. These components are associated with (1) wounds of Mr. X's left lower extremity resultant from vascular surgery, (2) a slow healing ulcer of his left ankle resultant from a minor impact, and (3) cellulitis and other effects of ischemic vascular disease of his left lower extremity. The nurse coordinates elements of the nursing system with Mr. X's vascular surgeon by communicating Mr. X's and her own observations and judgments. Mr. X coordinates components of his self-care system associated with his diabetes and his coronary artery disease and his pacemaker with his internist and cardiologist respectively. The nurse who bears and fulfills the responsibility for knowing the interactions among the health deviations as well as other components of Mr. X's therapeutic self-care demand acts to regulate such interactions in a positive fashion through advice and consultation to Mr. X and Mr. X's daughter-in-law.

SUMMARY

The three theories that together constitute the self-care deficit theory of nursing are structured by related conceptual elements that express the theory developers' understandings of what nursing is and what nursing can and should be. This theory explains that the professional, technological dimensions of nursing articulate with the social and interpersonal dimensions. Together they constitute a frame of reference for nursing practitioners and researchers as well as for continued theorizing about nursing.

A frame of reference is generally understood as a structure of concepts, values, and views by means of which an individual or group perceives or evaluates data, communicates ideas, and regulates behavior (Stein, 1973). Frames of reference are used in the sciences; for example, in physics they are used to organize observations and describe physical phenomena mathematically. In psychology two frames of reference have been traditionally used—the external or objective approach in which behavior is viewed and examined from an observer point of view and the personal, perceptual, or phenomenological approach in which observations are focused on how people see themselves.

Nurses who understand the self-care deficit theory of nursing view the professional, technological dimension of nursing within the conceptualizations in which the theory is expressed. They relate the professional, technological features of nursing to nursing's societal and interpersonal dimensions. They understand how the theories draw upon and synthesize relevant elements from the human sciences. They also understand that frames of reference from various human sciences must be known to nurses and used by them in making observations, evaluating data, and attaching meaning to data. For example, it is clear that when nurses view persons who seek and require nursing from the perspective of their self-care capabilities and the features of their usual systems of self-care they must use both of the frames of reference used by psychologists—the outside observer view and the personal or phenomenological view. The use of the broad nursing frame of reference provided by the three parts of the self-care deficit theory of nursing requires that nurses have knowledge of various human sciences including the concepts, values, and views by means of which data are perceived and evaluated. Frames within frames are characteristic of nursing theory as they are in all practice fields.

REFERENCES

Orem, D. E. (1985). *Nursing: Concepts of practice* (3rd ed.). New York: McGraw-Hill.

Orem, D. E., & Taylor, S. G. (1986). Orem's general theory of nursing. In P. Winstead-Fry (Ed.). *Case studies in nursing theory* (pp. 37–71). New York: National League for Nursing.

Stein, J. (Ed.). (1973). *The Random House dictionary of the English language.* New York: Random House.

Winstead-Fry (Ed.). (1986). *Case studies in nursing theory.* New York: National League for Nursing.

7

Practical Applications of Orem's Self-Care Deficit Nursing Theory

Susan G. Taylor

I have been asked to speak on "practical applications of SCDNT (Self-Care Deficit Nursing Theory)." Before beginning the substance of my presentation, I would like to clarify my interpretation of the word "practical." I take "practical" to mean "related to practice." I am not using the word in its more common usage of meaning concrete and useful as opposed to intellectual and esoteric. There is nothing simple or common sense about the use of nursing theory. It requires hard work and intellectual rigor to develop nursing practice methods from a nursing theory. Only after this kind of work has been done will we be able to talk of the practical in the colloquial sense.

Theory-based nursing has been defined as "nursing designed and produced for individuals and groups by nurses who have insights about and have conceptualized the specific characteristics of the human health service named nursing" (Orem, 1987). This definition suggests that there are at least two ways to approach nursing: the traditional approach and the theory-based approach. By the traditional approach I am referring to the approach that views nursing as what nurses do, to those practice activities that have been a part of the role of the nurse for some period of time and are accepted as legitimate nursing functions. Extension of practice activities in the traditional approach results from the practitioner's individual view of what constitutes legitimate practice. The practitioner may use a general model, such as General Systems Theory or development theory, to guide practice; but these models are not specific to nursing.

On the other hand, theory-based nursing occurs when the practitioner has taken the time and energy to conceptualize the object of nursing, the "human variables that are interactive in bringing about requirements for nursing, and the human variables that are interactive in the production of nursing in interpersonal or group situations" (Orem, 1987). Nursing practice is derived from the conceptualization and theory of nursing or when knowledge from other disciplines is brought into nursing by or through articulation with nursing theory.

Theory-based nursing has as its foundation a general theory of nursing that gives direction in gaining insights about nursing and guides decision making and action in nursing practice situations (Orem, 1987). The purpose of this presentation is to examine how one specific general theory of nursing, namely Orem's SCDNT, gives direction to nursing practice. This will be accomplished by looking at the use of the theory (1) at the individual practitioner level, (2) at the institutional level, and (3) in research and education. I will do this by presenting my views on the use of the theory and by giving examples of others' experiences with the use of the theory.

USE OF THEORY BY THE INDIVIDUAL PRACTITIONER

We all have and use a concept of nursing. For some it is an explicit formal model, while for others it is a developed personal implicit model. For the individual, the conceptual structure of nursing is developed first through the educational experiences of the nursing student. The way the student is taught to think about and conceptualize nursing sets the stage for the future practice. As a nurse, I have an established world view that forms the basis for my identification of problems, the way I look to resolve those problems, how I evaluate my outcomes, and the language I use to express my nursing judgments. For me, the essential aspect of theory-based nursing is the development by the individual practitioner of a way of thinking about or viewing the world of nursing that is based on an explicit theory or model. The advantages to using an explicit theoretical system include the validation of concepts, enhanced communication with other experts, and a valuing of common goals and objectives for care.

SCDNT provides me with the basis for determining who is a legitimate patient or client and for determining the essential parameters of nursing care requirements for such patients. For example, imagine working as a nurse in a clinic. Two patients have similar medical problems and have seen the physician for treatment of hypertension. As part of the protocol, all patients must check out with me after seeing the physician. How do I decide which of these patients needs to become a legitimate patient of the nurse? Mr. Jones has been given a new prescription. Mr. Smith is told to continue on his same regimen of drugs, diet, and activity. From the SCDNT perspective, I would begin by assessing the presence and nature of the existent self-care system and the effects and limitations of self-care on health. Mr. Jones is independent in his self-care, knows the general actions and expected effects of the new drug, and follows the previously prescribed diet; however, his blood pressure continues to be elevated. Mr. Smith, on the other hand, is dependent on his wife for his self-care. He assumes responsibility only for daily hygiene. He adheres to his diet and his drug regimen as long as Mrs. Smith provides the direction. They are both satisfied with the care system that they have established over the years. It is obvious that Mr. Smith has self-care limitations, even though his health care needs are being met and his blood pressure is under control, while Mr. Jones has fewer self-care limitations though his blood pressure is not under control.

Mr. Jones may need support in continuing to monitor his self-care and his response to certain life situations to further identify possible actions that could be taken to ameliorate the hypertension or to decrease the possibility of significant untoward effects. His primary problem is a medical one.

Mr. Smith may need to begin to assume some responsibility for his own care, at least to the extent of understanding what is happening to him and why the particular care measures have been prescribed. The extent to which this is done depends on his willingness and ability to learn and to take some responsibility as well as on his wife's willingness to share this responsibility. If Mr. Smith chooses not to participate in his own self-care, the nurse may want to work with Mrs. Smith to identify potential alternate care systems or resources for Mr. Smith in the event that she could not care for him.

Similarly, the nurse working in the hospital uses her knowledge of self-care and dependent care to make judgments about whether or not, from the nursing perspective, a patient is ready to be discharged from the hospital. The primary criterion used is the patient's ability to maintain or manage her or his own self-care or the existence of a support system—dependent care or professional nursing—that will be able to compensate for any limitations of self-care. If such systems are not available, the patient should be kept in the hospital or referred to a nursing home.

In both examples, the conceptual structure of the theory has given me the basis for assessment, for assigning meaning to the data perceived or collected, for thinking about the patient from a nursing perspective, and for communicating that process in a specific language. My ability to do this is not dependent on the setting in which I work. While I may be constrained in my use of the language system if I work in an agency that does not explicitly use the same model, my personal view of the meaning of data and of nursing does not need to change. I am able to maintain the nursing focus in my care.

There is no doubt that my use of theory is facilitated when there is compatibility between my personal view of nursing and that of the institution in which I practice. We have long admonished new practitioners to examine the philosophy of the nursing division before they take a position to ascertain that it is compatible with their own philosophy of nursing. This level of philosophical congruence is enhanced when the theoretical basis of practice is made explicit.

There are hundreds of nurses practicing from the perspective of SCDNT in this country and abroad. These nurses state that the use of the theory has helped them to be more focused and confident. They are able to clearly express the differences between nursing and other disciplines.

Two references listed in the bibliography may be of particular help in clarifying the use of the theory by the individual practitioner: Winstead-Fry's (1986) *Case Studies in Nursing Theory* and Taylor's (1988) article in *Nursing Science Quarterly*.

UNIT AND INSTITUTION-BASED NURSING

There are a number of instances where a unit within a hospital has decided to use SCDNT as the basis for nursing care in the unit, even though the hospital itself does not. The use of the theory provides a framework for common goals and objectives and congruent program practices. The basis for the development of a unit-based system is the description and identification of the characteristics of the populations being served on the unit from the perspective of the theory. This works well when units are decentralized and relatively independent.

The use of a common framework for an entire nursing division has many advantages. Besides the common focus and goals, there is consistency between the stated beliefs about nursing and the forms for recording and transmitting information about the process and outcomes of nursing. The process of developing an institution-wide theory-based nursing system is beyond the scope of this paper. When an institution decides to incorporate a theoretical approach to nursing, it will affect all levels of the organization including the philosophy, goals, and objectives; the standards and quality assurance program; and the documentation, job description, and personnel evaluation systems.

Example of Theory Use

I will now present an example of the use of SCDNT in a clinical situation.

I will begin by presenting brief excerpts from one institution's experience as an example of the internal consistency that results from the use of SCDNT.

Mission. In this example, the institution's mission is to create a nursing system that will facilitate patient ability to meet self-care requisites.

Philosophy. The institution's philosophy indicates that patients have primary responsibility for their self-care to the extent of their abilities. Patients exercise this responsibility through collaboration with the nursing staff in the development and implementation of the plan for care. Professional nurses bear responsibility and accountability for the delivery and documentation of the nursing care the patient receives.

Objectives. Institutional objectives are the following:

- To establish and maintain a practice model using SCDNT as the basis for defining nursing practice.
- To provide the patient the opportunity to collaborate with nursing in the development and implementation of a plan of care.
- To use all available resources to assist the patient and family in rehabilitation and continued care in the community.

For example, from the SCDNT perspective, the primary focus of the surgical clinical nurse specialist is on self-care demands arising from requisites to maintain processes of elimination and maintain skin integrity. The scope of practice encompasses nursing situations in which patients experience deficits in meeting these requisites. Roles and responsibilities include developing and implementing regulatory nursing systems for patients who have complex demands and/or whose demands require complex interventions, designing self-management systems for patients and families (care providers), and assisting nursing staff in developing patients' self-care abilities or their families' dependent care abilities.

From these brief excerpts, one can see that there is a consistent use of the language and the concepts of the theory in describing nursing. This consistency is seen also in the documentation of nursing, standards of care, and many other aspects of the delivery system.

Case Study

I will conclude this section with a short case study and projected nursing system design to illustrate the use of SCDNT.

Mr. Brown, 64 years of age, was admitted to the hospital for acute exacerbation of chronic obstructive pulmonary disease with respiratory failure. He had a long history of smoking, though he had quit three years ago. He lives alone and would walk to town for lunch every day. He has one son who lives nearby and a daughter living several hundred miles away. Prior to admission he was on oral theophylline and inhaled bronchodilators.

On admission, Mr. Brown was alert but in severe respiratory distress. He was treated with IV theophylline, high dose steroids, antibiotics, high flow nebulizer, and low flow oxygen. His condition improved within 24 hours so that intubation was not necessary. His hospital stay lasted eight days, after which he was discharged to his home with instructions for use of one liter of oxygen per nasal cannula, high flow nebulization treatments, and medications.

A home nursing referral was made. Instructions included making sure that he used his nebulizer and oxygen correctly, reviewing his medication schedule with him, and perhaps setting aside the correct doses for him. The home health nurse was asked to assess his lung function and exercise routine. When the nurse made her first visit, Mr. Brown announced that he no longer would be making his daily trip to town for lunch and that he intended to sit in his rocking chair "for the rest of his days." He told her that if he needed oxygen he must be too sick to do anything else and besides he couldn't go anywhere if he had to have oxygen.

Nursing System Developed for Mr. Brown. Mr. Brown's particularized self-care requisites are defined as the following:

- Maintain oxygen exchange optimally, within limits of tolerance for exercise, using oxygen, high flow nebulization, and medications.
- Increase tolerance for exercise or maintain present level.

- Know how to manage home oxygen.
- Understand the function and use of oxygen, including safety precautions and whom to contact for assistance.
- Maintain adequate hydration and nutrition with high Vitamin C content fluids.
- Monitor pulmonary function using Flowmeter.
- Reestablish social interactions by having visitors and attending social functions.
- Avoid social contact with persons who have upper respiratory infections.
- Monitor elimination for changes from normal (e.g., constipation due to reduced activity) and take action to relieve or prevent difficulties.
- Control expenditure of energy to accomplish necessary tasks such as bathing and general hygiene.
- Develop a realistic image of capabilities, limitations, and potential for change.
- Develop a satisfying life pattern within limitations.
- Know and monitor effectiveness of medications and watch for side effects.

Mr. Brown has the following capabilities:

- Aptitude for manual activities.
- Alert and oriented.
- Able to manage usual self-care system satisfactorily.
- Accepting of professional help.

Mr. Brown has the following limitations:

- No antecedent knowledge or experience related to managing oxygen equipment.
- Limited family support system.
- No data available regarding most of the foundational capabilities and dispositions, power components, or basic conditioning factors.

Because of the limited data, the following nursing diagnoses are tentative:

- Lack of knowledge of appropriate actions to meet new demands.
- Inability to accept limitations imposed by new demands.
- Insufficient energy to provide all aspects of self-care.
- Decreased motivation to care for self.

The nursing action plan consists of the following:

- Assess and monitor status of self-care requisites. (Are they being met fully, partially, not at all, inappropriately, or unsatisfactorily?)
- Do detailed nursing history and assessment regarding self-care agency.
- Clarify basis for response to requirement for oxygen therapy and other limitations.
- Develop further plans.

USE IN EDUCATION AND RESEARCH

In discussing the use of theory, it is important to mention the value of theory to research and education. Because of the limit of time, I will only bring this to your attention. For detailed discussions of these topics, refer to Riehl-Sisca's (1985) *The Science and Art of Self-Care* and monographs available from the University of Missouri-Columbia School of Nursing, Continuing Education program.

REFERENCES

Orem, D. (1985). *Nursing: Concepts of practice.* (3rd ed.). New York: McGraw-Hill.

Orem, D. (1987). Why theory-based nursing? In S. Taylor, & E. Geden (Eds.). *Theory-based nursing process and product: Using Orem's SCDNT in practice, education and research.* Paper presented at the Fifth Annual SCDNT Conference, University of Missouri-Columbia.

Orem, D., & Taylor, S. (1988). Orem's general theory of nursing. In P. Winstead-Fry (Ed.). *Case studies in nursing theory.* New York: National League for Nursing.

Taylor, S.G. (1988). Nursing theory and nursing process. *Nursing Science Quarterly, 1* (3), 111–119.

Taylor, S.G. (1985). Teaching self-care deficit theory to generic students: Structuring pre-service curriculum. In J. Riehl-Sisca (Ed.): *The science and art of self-care.* New York: Appleton-Century-Crofts.

Taylor, S.G. (Ed.). (1988). *Nursing agency and nursing systems.* Paper presented at the Sixth Annual SCDNT Conference, University of Missouri-Columbia.

Winstead-Fry, P. (1986). *Case studies in nursing theory.* New York: National League for Nursing.

Part 4

King's Theory of Goal Attainment

8

King's Conceptual Framework and Theory of Goal Attainment

Imogene M. King

Within the past 15 years, many articles about philosophies of science, theory, research, and the relationships among these ideas have appeared in the nursing literature (Chinn, 1983; Fawcett & Downs, 1986; Hardy, 1978; Silva, 1977 & 1984; Suppe & Jacox, 1985). In addition, several books have presented critiques of published theoretical positions (Fawcett, 1989; Marriner-Tomey, 1989). Some of these writings indicate that nurse theorists have been influenced by the traditional scientific mode called the "received view" by some and "reductionism" by others.

Because my initial orientation to research was qualitative, I questioned many of the studies that reported two variables and used a quasi-experimental design to study nursing. The complexity and variety in nursing situations can hardly be reduced to two variables. Somehow the critical variables were not always identified in the early studies. I kept looking for, and finally found, a philosophical orientation to science that was congruent with my philosophy of nursing. That philosophical orientation was General System Theory.

General System Theory was given prominence with the (1956) General System Theory yearbook. Three articles in that edition presented the basic concepts and elements of this movement (Fagan & Hall, Von Bertalanffy, & Boulding). Von Bertalanffy, often called the father of General System Theory, expanded the basic ideas in a book published in 1968. He defined the scientific approach taken by General System Theory as "perspectivism" as opposed to the traditional scientific mode of reductionism. He also noted that General System Theory is the science of wholeness. So, please, all of you "critiquers," read my conceptual framework and Theory of Goal Attainment from the perspective of General System Theory and a science of wholeness, which is my philosophical position. After studying the research on General System Theory, I was able to synthesize my analysis of the nursing literature and my knowledge from other disciplines into a conceptual framework.

My inquiry into the essence of professional nursing began with a few questions. What is nursing? Who is a nurse? What functions do nurses perform as professionals? Where do they perform their functions? What is a nursing act? What is the nursing process? Following a review of nursing literature and my experiences as a nurse and as a teacher of nursing students, I began to find information to help me answer some of these questions and to ask more questions.

My conceptual framework was published in 1971 in a book called *Toward a Theory for Nursing*. This framework, composed of concepts derived from my review of nursing literature, provided the structure for me to continue my review of the research literature related to the concepts. Indeed, one purpose of a conceptual framework is to guide the construction of theory in a discipline.

KING'S CONCEPTUAL FRAMEWORK

A conceptual framework based on General System Theory was proposed to provide a comprehensive view of the three dynamic interacting systems that form the environments that influence individuals' growth, development, work, and death. Figure 8-1 illustrates the interaction of these three systems: the personal

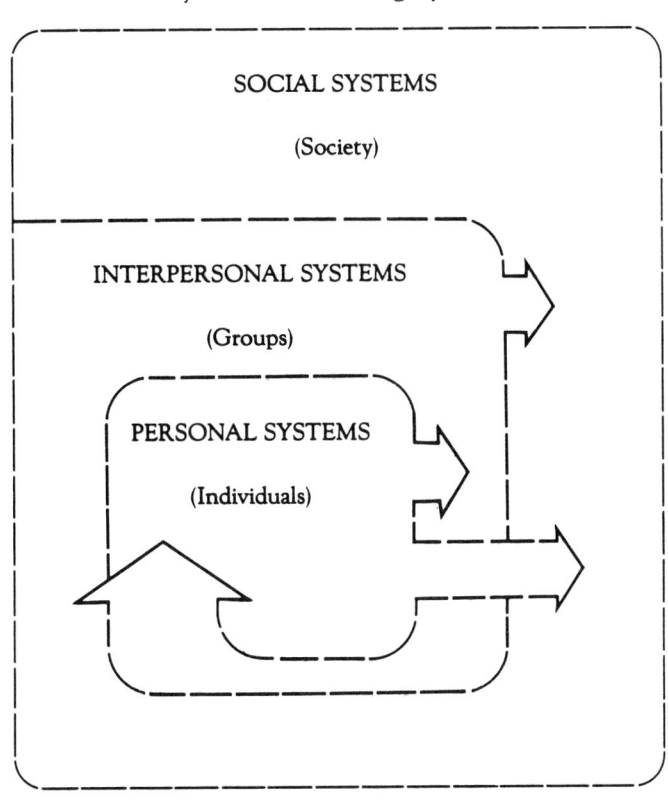

Figure 8-1
Dynamic Interacting Systems

SOCIAL SYSTEMS

(Society)

INTERPERSONAL SYSTEMS

(Groups)

PERSONAL SYSTEMS

(Individuals)

Reprinted from King, I.M. (1981). *A Theory for Nursing: Systems, Process, Concepts*, p. 11. New York: Delmar Publishers, Inc.. Reprinted by permission.

(individuals), interpersonal (dyads, triads, and groups), and social (institutions and organizations). One purpose of this framework is to identify concepts that are essential knowledge for nursing as a discipline. The concepts identified in nursing's literature cut across many disciplines. A second purpose of this framework is to construct and test theories from the perspective of a specific discipline, which in this instance is nursing.

Five essential elements of each system are goal(s), structure, functions, resources, and decision making. Using these elements as criteria, my conceptual framework has health as the *goal* for nursing. Health is defined conceptually from a review of the literature in a variety of disciplines as "dynamic life experiences of a human being, which implies continuous adjustment to stressors in the internal and external environment through optimum use of one's resources to achieve maximum potential for daily living" (King, 1981). Health is perceived as an individual's ability to function in one's usual roles.

The *structure* of my framework is composed of three open systems of persons interacting with the environment. The *functions* of these three systems (personal, individual, and social) are identified in the reciprocal relations of individuals as they interact in groups such as families and communities. For example, maintaining the nutritional status of individuals in families will influence behavior in the educational system, in the health care system, and in the work system. *Resources* are essential to keep the three systems in harmony and balance. Two major categories of resources are people, such as health professionals and clients, and money, which provides equipment and supplies to carry out specific functions. *Decision making* is a critical element in any system in which choices must be made in order to allocate resources to perform the functions and attain the goals of the system. In my thinking, a General System approach to developing a conceptual framework for nursing was the natural approach to take in developing theories for nursing because General System Theory is a science of wholeness, as is nursing.

From my conceptual framework, a Theory of Goal Attainment was derived. This is a General System Theory of the human interaction process that leads to transactions that in turn lead to goal attainment.

KING'S THEORY OF GOAL ATTAINMENT

When a theory is formulated from a specific conceptual framework, some of the same concepts used to develop the framework provide substantive knowledge about the theory. In order to explicate the philosophical assumptions of the Theory of Goal

Attainment, I will list *my philosophical assumptions* about human beings:

- Individuals are social beings.
- Individuals are sentient beings.
- Individuals are rational beings.
- Individuals are reacting beings.
- Individuals are perceiving beings.
- Individuals are controlling beings.
- Individuals are purposeful beings.
- Individuals are action-oriented beings.
- Individuals are time-oriented beings (King, 1981).

One assumption from the original work was omitted in this paper, and that is that "individuals are spiritual beings."→

Since the components of the Theory of Goal Attainment relate to two or more individuals interacting in a nursing situation, specific assumptions about nurse and client interactions are explicated as follows:

- Perceptions of nurse and of client influence the interaction process.
- Goals, needs, and values of nurse and client influence the interaction process.
- Individuals have a right to knowledge about themselves.
- Individuals have a right to participate in decisions that influence their life, their health, and community services.
- Health professionals have a responsibility to share information that helps individuals make informed decisions about their health care.
- Individuals have a right to accept or reject health care.
- Goals of health professionals and goals of recipients of health care may be incongruent (King, 1981).

This personal philosophy of human beings and of human interactions between nurse and client influenced the development of my conceptual framework and Theory of Goal Attainment.

CONCEPTS

Ten concepts from the conceptual framework were selected as the major concepts of the Theory of Goal Attainment:

- Perception
- Communication
- Interaction
- Transaction
- Self
- Role
- Growth and Development
- Time
- Personal Space
- Stress

All of these concepts are defined from a review of research and theoretical literature (King, 1981). One concept, transaction, has been operationally defined which provides a classification system of interactions that lead to transactions and thus to goal attainment. A descriptive study was conducted to observe the behaviors in nurse-patient interactions. Interaction data from two separate studies were used to confirm the presence of transactions in nurse-patient interactions. A model of nurse-patient transaction is shown in figure 8-2.

When two individuals come together in any situation, each is perceiving the other, making mental judgments, taking some mental action, and reacting. One cannot directly observe these behaviors, but one can directly observe verbal and nonverbal behavior and record the interactions to analyze for transactions. Nurse-patient interactions can be classified into the following categories:

- Action
- Reaction
- Disturbance
- Mutual goal setting

Figure 8-2
A Model of Transaction

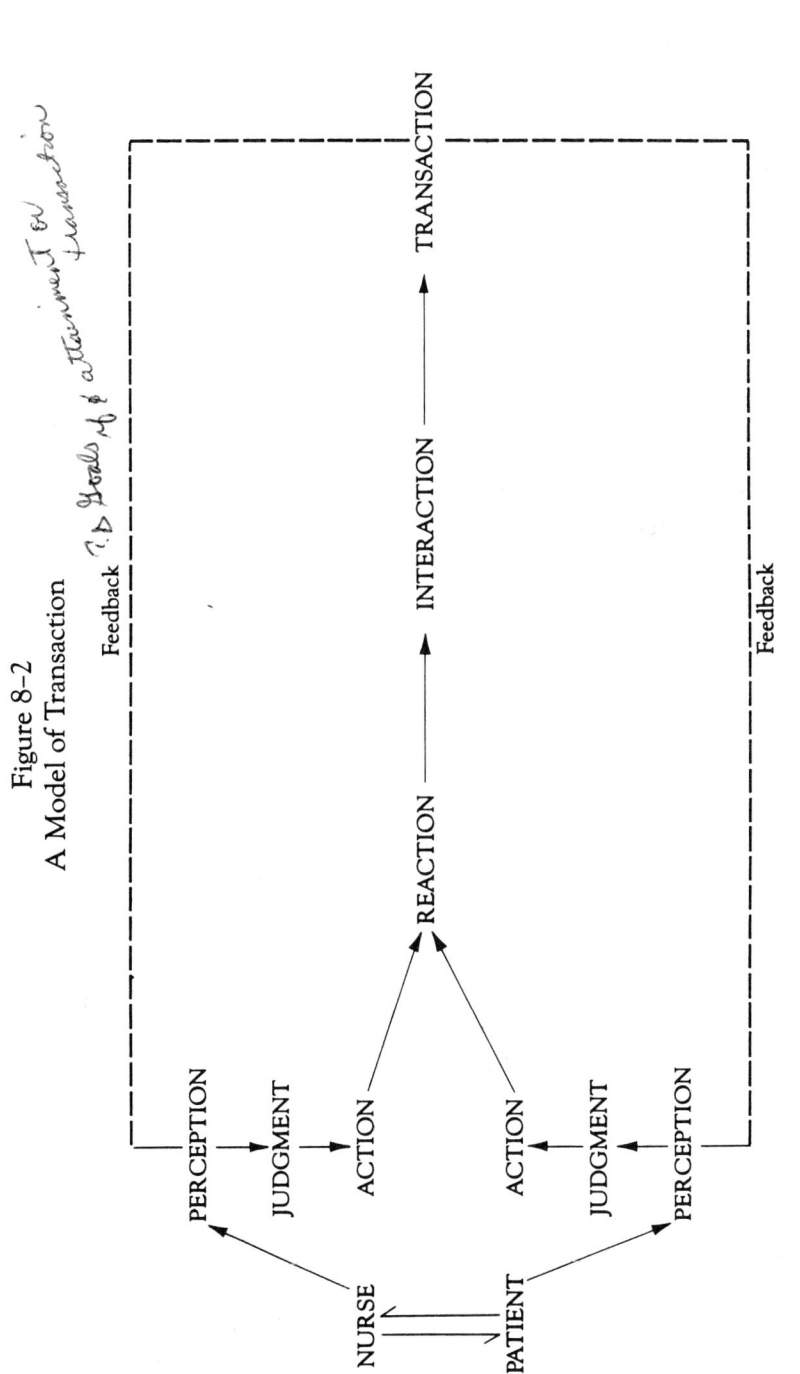

Feedback → Goals of attainment &r transaction

```
PERCEPTION → JUDGMENT → ACTION
                                  ↘
NURSE ↗                             REACTION → INTERACTION → TRANSACTION
      ⇄                           ↗
PATIENT ↘                       
         PERCEPTION ← JUDGMENT ← ACTION
```

Feedback

Reprinted from King, I. M. (1981). *A Theory for Nursing: Systems Concepts and Process*, p. 145. New York: Delmar Publishers, Inc. Reprinted by permission.

- Exploration of means to achieve goal
- Agreement on means to achieve goal
- Transaction
- Attainment of goal (King, 1981).

From the results of this descriptive study, my definition of nursing was formulated: "Nursing is a process of human interactions between nurse and client whereby each person perceives the other and the situation, and through communication they set goals, explore means, and agree on means to achieve goals" (King, 1981). Both individuals exhibit behaviors that show movement toward goal attainment. One criterion for evaluating a theory is to determine if there are relations among the concepts. Propositional statements indicate these relations (King, 1981). Figure 8–3 shows relationships among the concepts as specified by the following propositions:

- Perceptual accuracy, role congruence, and communication in a nurse-client interaction leads to transactions.

Figure 8–3
Relationship Between Role Conflict and Stress

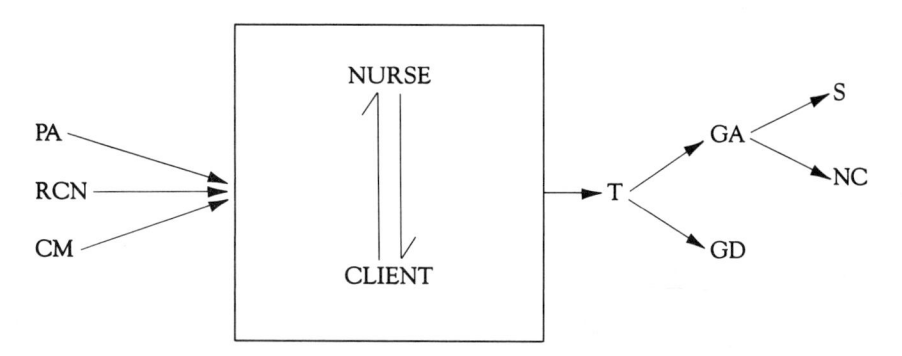

Note: Perceptual accuracy (PA); Role congruence (RCN); Communication (CM); Transaction (T); Goal attainment (GA); Growth and development (GD); Satisfaction (S); Effective nursing care (NC).
Adapted from Austin, J., & Champion V. (1983). King's theory for nursing: Explication and evaluation. In P. Chinn (Ed.). *Advances in Nursing Theory Development* (p. 54). Rockville, MD: Aspen.

King's Framework & Theory

- Transactions lead to goal attainment and growth and development.
- Goal attainment leads to satisfaction and to effective nursing care.

Two nurses who critiqued my theory also diagrammed relations among my concepts as stated in the propositions (Austin & Champion, 1983).

Figure 8-4 shows the relationships specified by the proposition "Role conflict in nurse-client interactions leads to stress."

One purpose of a theory is to generate research questions or to state testable hypotheses. The following hypotheses are examples of several being tested this year:

- Mutual goal setting will increase ability to perform activities of daily living.
- Mutual goal setting by nurse and patient leads to goal attainment.
- Goal attainment will be greater in patients who participate in goal setting than those who do not participate in goal setting.

Figure 8-4
Relationship Among Concepts in the Theory of Goal Attainment

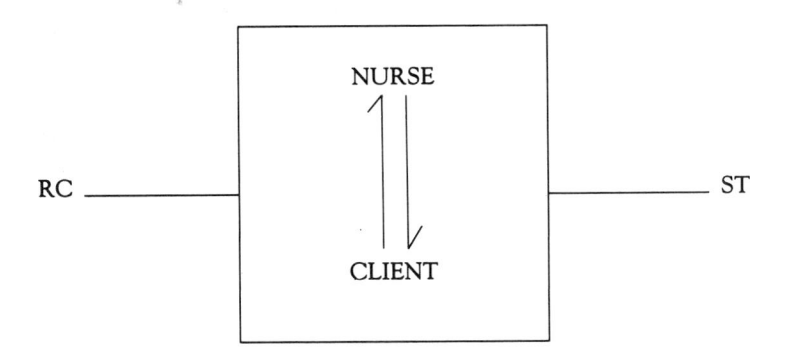

```
            ┌─────────────┐
            │   NURSE     │
            │    ↑│       │
    RC ─────┤    ││       ├───── ST
            │    │↓       │
            │   CLIENT    │
            └─────────────┘
```

Note: Role conflict (RC); Stress (ST).
Adapted from Austin, J., & Champion V. (1983). King's theory for nursing: Explication and evaluation. In P. Chinn (Ed.). *Advances in Nursing Theory Development* (p. 54). Rockville, MD: Aspen.

- Mutual goal setting will increase elderly patients' morale.
- Perceptual congruence in nurse-patient interactions increases mutual goal setting.
- Goal attainment decreases stress and anxiety in nursing situations.
- Congruence in role expectations and role performance increases transactions in nurse-patient interactions.

My theory is that nursing is a process of interactions that lead to transactions. Transactions lead to goal attainment. Goal attainment is a measure of effective nursing care. The model of transactions shown in figure 8-2 provides a theoretical basis for the nursing process as method (table 8-1).

To implement the Theory of Goal Attainment in practice, a Goal-Oriented Nursing Record was proposed (King, 1981). This documentation system was operationalized for use in dialysis units (King, 1984). It consists of a nursing data base that assesses patient abilities to perform activities of daily living. Information is gathered about the role of the patient prior to hospitalization and about the patient's and family's perceptions of the health concerns. The

Table 8-1
Nursing Process

Nursing Process as Method	Nursing Process as Theory
A system of interrelated actions	A system of interrelated concepts
Assess	Perception of nurse and client Communication of nurse and client Interaction of nurse and client
Plan	Decision making about goals Explore means to attain goals Agree to means to attain goals
Implement	Transactions made
Evaluate	Goal attained (if not, why not)?

Source for method: Yura, H., & Walsh, M. (1983) *The nursing process.* CT: Appleton-Century-Crofts.
Source for theory: King, I.M. (1981) *A theory for nursing: Systems, process and concepts.* NY: John Wiley & Sons.

nurse assesses knowledge about the patient's learning needs. From this data base, nursing diagnoses are recorded. Goals are mutually set with patients when possible. In these interactions, nurses give patients information to help them make informed decisions. Patients give nurses information that helps nurses gather relevant information. From the goal list, which has identified the behavioral outcomes expected for patients, nursing orders are written. When goals have been identified and the progress notes indicate that the goals have been attained, a measure of effective nursing care has been documented.

RESEARCH

Studies are being conducted to test hypotheses generated from the concepts of the Theory of Goal Attainment. Several nurses have been deriving theories from my conceptual framework (Frey, 1989).

PRACTICE

Several hospitals in North America have implemented theory-based practice using my conceptual framework, Theory of Goal Attainment, and Goal-Oriented Nursing Record system. The most recent innovation is to use my conceptual framework as the structure for a quality assurance program with the Theory of Goal Attainment as the process for a quality assurance program and the Goal-Oriented Nursing Record system as the documentation system to record patient outcomes.

REFERENCES

Austin, J. K., & Champion, V. L. (1983). King's theory for nursing: Explication and evaluation. In P. Chinn, (Ed.). *Advances in nursing theory development* (pp. 45–61). Rockville, MD: Aspen.

Boulding, K. (1956). General systems theory—The skeleton of science. *Yearbook of the Society for the Advancement of General System Theory, 1*(1), 11–17.

Chinn, P. & Jacobs, M. (1983). *Theory and nursing.* St. Louis, MO: C.V. Mosby.

Fawcett, J. (1989). *Analysis and evaluation of conceptual models in nursing.* Philadelphia, PA: F. A. Davis.

Fawcett, J., & Downs, F. S. (1986). *The relationship between theory and research.* Norwalk, CT: Appleton-Century-Crofts.

Frey, M. A. (1989). Social support and health: A theoretical formulation derived from King's conceptual framework. *Nursing Science Quarterly, 2*(3), 138–148.

Hall, A. D., & Fagan, R. E. (1956). Definition of system. *Yearbook of the Society for the Advancement of General System Theory, 1*(1), 18–28.

Hardy, M. E. (1978). Perspectives on nursing theory. *Advances in Nursing Science, 1*(1).

King, I. M. (1971). *Toward a theory for nursing.* New York: John Wiley & Sons.

King, I. M. (1981). *A theory for nursing: Systems, process, concepts.* Albany, NY: Delmar Publications.

King, I. M. (1984). Effective measure of nursing: Use of King's goal oriented nursing record in renal dialysis units. *American Association of Nephrology Nurses and Technicians, 11*(2), 11.

Marriner-Tomey, A. (1989). *Nursing theorists and their work.* St. Louis, MO: C. V. Mosby.

Silva, M. C. (1977). Philosophy, science, theory: Interrelationships and implications for nursing research. *Image, 9*(3).

Silva, M. C., & Rothbart, D. (1984). An analysis of changing trends in philosophies of science on nursing theory development and testing. *Advances in Nursing Science, 7*(1).

Suppe, F., & Jacox, A. K. (1985). Philosophy of science and the development of nursing theory. In H. Werley & J. Fitspatrick (Eds.). *Annual Review of Nursing Research,* Vol. 3. New York: Springer Publishers.

Von Bertalanffy, L. (1956). General system theory. *Yearbook of the Society for the Advancement of General Systems Theory, 1*(1), 1–10.

Von Bertalanffy, L. (1968). *General system theory.* New York: George Braziller.

9

Implementing King's Conceptual Framework at the Bedside

*Esther Byrne Coker and
Rita Schreiber*

The challenge in implementing a conceptual framework is to do it in a way that is meaningful and useful to the nurses at the bedside. This is what faced our nursing department in 1984 when our move to theory-based practice began.

When this whole process was begun, we would not have pictured it working out the way it has. When we first began thinking about implementing a conceptual framework, there was little written about how to do it. Of course, there were the theories and conceptual frameworks themselves, and an increasing amount of research based on them, but people were not yet writing about how they used theory as a basis for real-life clinical practice. So we struggled somewhat blindly. It has worked out well, although perhaps not quite as it was planned. Our biggest lesson has been that one cannot make concrete plans at the outset. It has been to our advantage to be open to the opportunities that happen by chance.

This paper will begin with a brief history—how and why we chose a conceptual framework, and King's in particular. We will then discuss how we in the nursing department thought we should go about implementing theory-based practice. Following this, we will present the actual strategies we used. We will conclude with a brief look into the future.

BACKGROUND

The College of Nurses of Ontario has proposed a new set of standards for practice. Contained within these standards is reference to the fact that nurses should be practicing from a theoretical base. This belief has been the impetus for many hospitals to begin looking for a conceptual framework.

At Centenary Hospital about six years ago, in preparation for choosing a framework, nurses began to examine their assumptions and beliefs about their practice. This was a long and arduous process, involving much soul searching. Nurses from all levels of practice and all areas of the hospital comprised what was then known as the Nursing Quality Assurance Committee. The nurses began examining the works of various nursing theorists, looking for a conceptual framework that had an assumptive base similar to their own. The nurses at Centenary Hospital felt the conceptual framework of Imogene King was the best fit.

Choosing the framework was just the beginning. The next step was to figure out how to implement it. There was a great deal we did not know, but there were a few things that we *did* know. To begin with, the plan was to have the conceptual framework fully operational throughout the hospital within three years.

Members of the Nursing Quality Assurance Committee knew they wanted to begin by focusing on King's Conceptual Framework rather than her Theory of Goal Attainment. They thought a logical place to begin with was the assessment phase of the nursing process. To do this, the prototype of a Nursing History and Assessment Record based on King's Conceptual Framework was devised by members of the committee. This tool was designed to assist nurses in becoming familiar with the framework while gathering assessment data based on the framework. As can be imagined, this too was a massive undertaking. It can be appreciated that when a group of about 20 nurses get together with their own interests at heart, no stone will be left unturned. What resulted was a 23-page document which put chills up peoples' spines! The nursing department quickly realized that no single assessment form would suit the needs of all clinical areas. It would be up to each clinical area to revise the form in such a way that it would meet their specific needs.

Rather than using pilot units for implementation of the framework, each nursing directorate was to proceed in its own style, at its own pace. This is where the implementation story at the directorate level really begins.

BEGINNING

Our directorate at that time was the Continuing Care directorate. It included three gerontology units, a rehabilitation unit, and a psychiatry unit. Nursing managers from these clinical units met regularly with the clinical nurse specialist and the clinical instructor. The directorate has recently expanded to include the emergency department and the orthopedic unit and is now called the Specialty Services directorate.

We, as other directorates, spent a great deal of time scratching our heads and saying, "Great! Now what?" At countless meetings we read excerpts from King's book, discussed application of her theory, and struggled to prepare ourselves to "spread the word." We lived in constant fear of how we would handle difficult questions and/or resistance. As we struggled, we formulated some guiding principles. At least we knew what we didn't want.

We did not want theory-based practice to seem threatening. We did not want nurses to feel that anyone was criticizing their current practice. We wanted to remove the fog of mystification that so often puts nursing theory into an ivory tower quite far from the nurse at the bedside. We did not want it to be viewed as impractical. We wanted to be able to answer the question in every nurse's mind (if not on her lips): "What's in it for us?"

We did not want the implementation to be viewed as just another massive project for already overworked nurses. We wanted them to see that theory-based practice was not separate from their daily nursing practice, but that it was just a way of reflecting on their practice and talking about it.

We knew enough not to expect instant conversion. We expected it to be a slow process. We sought to raise people's awareness of the systems and concepts of the framework and how they applied to daily nursing practice. We did not want nurses to reject the idea of theory-based practice just because it would not solve many of the problems they felt were of concern at the time. We felt that if they had a realistic view of what a conceptual framework could and could not do for them, they would not be likely to reject it because it failed to meet their expectations.

It was at this point that we decided to stop talking about it and take the plunge. We decided to risk learning right along with the rest of the staff nurses and admit that we weren't the experts. This courageous feat was well worth it. As the first directorate in the hospital to get moving, we're now the furthest along, and we're now beginning to see the fruits of our labors.

STRATEGIES

Not long after the decision to adopt King's Conceptual Framework was made, the Nursing department, in cooperation with our Training and Development department, revised the general nursing orientation in such a way that it reflected the framework. During orientation we focus on the nurse's *Personal System;* we give nurses the opportunity to discuss their values and compare them with those of the hospital. We look at the nurse's new *Social System,* which is Centenary Hospital, and discuss how we define the role of the nurse. We then move into the nurse's *Interpersonal System,* where we teach them how to use themselves effectively by practicing communication skills. At this point in the orientation they also meet representatives from other departments such as the pharmacy and supply services.

Later in the orientation, we focus on the patient's *Interpersonal System,* and look at how we work with patients. The tasks of the nursing process are presented in relation to the overall goals and direction of Centenary nursing. We emphasize interpersonal relationships by following a fictitious patient from admission to discharge. Nurses also have an opportunity to meet with other professionals who work with our patients, for example, physicians, occupational therapists, and chaplains.

At the end of the orientation program, we formally teach King's framework and show the new employees how they have already been using the framework throughout the week. By this time, people are ready to accept the framework because they have seen how their own practice relates to our chosen framework. Through discussion, nurses new to Centenary begin to see the usefulness of King's Conceptual Framework in their daily practice. To further the process, specific clinical areas have devised unit orientations that are natural extensions of the general nursing orientation and are based on the systems and concepts outlined by King. By the end of the two-week orientation period, new nurses have received the message loud and clear that we take theory-based practice seriously.

To begin the process of familiarizing nurses with King's Conceptual Framework, hospital-wide educational sessions were offered soon after the framework was chosen. These sessions, which were held on all shifts, introduced nurses to King's concepts and systems. To further the process in our directorate, we conducted educational sessions specific to each clinical area. These 45-minute inservice sessions were offered until every staff nurse in the directorate was able to attend. The content included an overview of conceptual frameworks and theory development as well as a description of King's three systems and 16 concepts. We spent some time discussing each concept in light of our own clinical areas; for example, our gerontology nurses were quick to point out that for some of their patients the use of touch was helpful and for others it was seen as an invasion of privacy. These differences between clients could be understood in the context of King's concept of *personal space* and all its facets.

Around this time, we provided a series of topical presentations for nurses working in psychiatry and gerontology. The assessment phase of the nursing process was highlighted in psychiatry by a series entitled "Assessment à la King." The gerontology nurses learned about assessment of the older adult. King's concepts were highlighted throughout these presentations.

We knew that merely presenting inservice sessions would not be sufficient to help nurses learn to incorporate King into their practice. The sessions were informative, but we had no idea how much was sinking in. One day while we and our unit managers were scratching our heads, thinking how overwhelming this was for us and how *very* overwhelming it must be for the staff nurses, someone had an idea. We wanted to make this formidable task of implementing the framework a manageable one. We decided to attack it piece by piece, or concept by concept, as it turned out. We thought that learning about one concept each month would be manageable. Since we wanted the nurses to be able to apply the concepts to their care, we came up with the following exercise. Each month, a concept was featured and information about the concept, taken from King's text, was posted. In addition, mini-discussions, 15 minutes each, highlighted the selected concept and encouraged nurses to begin thinking about it. Nurses thought about how the concept influenced their nursing care that particular month and were asked to write this on the perimeter of the poster. This helped stimulate others' ideas and promoted discussion about actual nursing care in the context of King's framework. That was what we had hoped for. This exercise carried on for 16 months and was fondly referred to as, "Concept of the Month."

This project was far more successful than any of us could have predicted. Although we set it up, *the nurses were the ones to actually apply* King's framework. We would like to share with you some examples of how our nurses believed King's ideas were useful. Before we do that, however, we will briefly describe King's Conceptual Framework for Nursing Practice.

King describes the practice of nursing as taking place within three dynamic interacting systems: Personal Systems, Interpersonal Systems, and Social Systems. The framework indicates that the focus of nursing is the care of human beings. It offers a framework of knowledge which allows the nurses to see the client as a total person reacting to his or her environment, taking into consideration the influence of his or her past, his or her present situation, and his or her goals for the future. The framework focuses not only on the client, but also on the nurse, providing direction in relation to his or her responsibility to the community and to the profession. The goal of this framework is the health of individuals, groups, and society.

After each of the following examples, we will explain which aspect of the framework the nurse was operationalizing. We'll begin with a look at the Personal System. Personal Systems are those that involve the individual. Each human being makes up a total system of his or her own. The nurse, then, is a total system, as is the client. King suggests that knowledge about the following six concepts will allow the nurse to more effectively assess and identify present or potential health problems, that is, to make accurate nursing diagnoses. Presented below is a sample of the comments made by the nurses with regard to the concepts of the Personal System.

The Personal System

Perception. "A family member of a patient overheard staff comments, but just one aspect of the conversation, and misunderstood the whole situation. Therefore, her perception of the situation can be considered unrealistic or misconstrued." A group of individuals may observe the same event but each person perceives it differently. This nurse identified that when a perceptual gap exists between caregivers and family members, misunderstandings occur.

Self. "Miss L.'s feelings of self-esteem are low; she is angry and bitter, possibly related to the losses and perceived injustices in her growing-up years. She has been dehumanized by chronic pain and long-term institutionalization. Her anger and low feelings of self-worth are reflected in her attitudes and behaviors toward us. We need to work on her feelings of self-esteem and perhaps may see reflected positive attitudes toward us." This nurse understood Miss L.'s inner world and realized that dehumanization and depersonalization can occur as a client enters the health care system. This nurse has been able to explain the reasons for this patient's behavior in the context of the concept of self. Her proposed nursing interventions show that she understood the problem behavior as stemming from low self-esteem.

Body Image. "A manic patient, who had gained quite a bit of weight since her last admission, came to a therapy group and told both patients and staff how 'fat' they were getting while she was 'losing weight.' She was projecting a distorted body image and displacing her anger." This nurse recognized how a disturbed body image can be reflected in a person's behavior.

"Mr. P. had a bad accident and now has an altered body image. He and his family are having a hard time accepting this and we as nurses must help them through this difficult time in their lives. We need to give the family and patient room to express their thoughts and feelings and encourage them to observe the wound, and answer the many questions they may have. Due to their culture, this will affect the entire family and if we can have one family member accept the situation, they can maybe help the other family members." The nurse recognized what King says about nurses needing to help patients maintain self-esteem when there is a distortion in body image. King also says that family members may need help from nurses to cope with changes in the body image of a loved one because the patient may be watching responses from family members to detect acceptance, rejection, pity, or anger. The nurse was also quick to note the influence of sociocultural factors on body image.

Growth and Development. "Mr. M. is 16 years old and is in Erikson's stage of Identity vs. Role Diffusion. The patient attempts to socialize and be accepted by older patients that he looks up to. He seems at times to act in a mature manner—at other times he seems to regress to a more immature level. The patient is given positive reinforcement when appropriately behaving, but limits are set (ie., privileges revoked) for inappropriate behavior such as the reckless use of his wheelchair." King says that behavior can sometimes be understood if the nurse has some knowledge of a client's background of growth and development. This nurse realized that this type of behavior is typical of a teenager cooped up in a hospital and geared her interventions accordingly.

Time. "Sometimes we as nurses are so busy that half an hour may pass before we get back to a patient we promised we would return to in ten minutes. To a patient lying in bed waiting for a nurse to perform a procedure or give an analgesic, it can seem like an hour." This nurse was sympathetic to what King says about time—that one person may perceive the same period of time as longer in duration than another person because of the various kinds of events in which the person is involved. Waiting makes the time seem long, and sensory deprivation may distort people's time perception. This nurse recognizes that time goes more slowly for patients than for herself and she understands the importance of following through with promises.

Space. "My patient is schizophrenic and needs his space. He likes no one behind him moving through a doorway. I moved a chair to be closer to interview him. He got up and placed the chair back in the original position farther away." This nurse was aware of some of the characteristics of space. It is situational in that each situation changes the need for and the way one uses space. It is also transactional—the way in which people perceive space influences the way they will behave in certain spatial situations. The nurse's knowledge of the concept of space helped her to understand her patient's behavior and allowed her to adjust her care accordingly.

The importance of space in the following example is self-evident:

"When patients have their curtains drawn or their doors closed, the nurse, doctor, and hospital personnel feel they have the liberty to walk in without knocking. We as professionals must think about how this makes a patient feel, and put ourselves in their shoes. Personally, I would like my privacy respected. We must all try to be more receptive to the needs of the patient." Dr. King says that space is often violated by hospital personnel, sometimes without asking permission. This nurse realized how important personal space is for patients and saw a need for a change in the way we approach patients in their rooms.

Next we will discuss the Interpersonal System. In King's framework, emphasis is placed on human beings who function in several types of interpersonal systems, that is, in dyads, triads, or groups. As the number of individuals increases, the complexity of the interaction increases. The following are examples of nurses' comments in regard to each concept in the Interpersonal System.

The Interpersonal System

Interaction. "As nurses and patients have increased interactions, positive and/or negative reactions can be observed. With more frequent interactions, there is greater opportunity for trust to develop." Interactions, according to King, are the acts of two or more persons in mutual presence. Interactions can reveal how one person thinks and feels about another person, how each perceives the other and what the other does to him, what his expectations are of the other, and how each reacts to the actions of the other. This nurse saw the importance of *every* interaction with a patient in that it helps to build the relationship between the patient and nurse.

Communication. "Mr. C. has had a hard time interpreting verbal and written communication and is, therefore, very frustrated. He demonstrates this with both verbal and nonverbal actions. Nursing care helps decrease patient frustrations by using simple sentences or single words. We also interpret his sign language, eg., pointing out what he wants if he's not able to state it verbally." These nurses have found ways to allow for the effective exchange of information, despite the patient's limitations.

Transaction. "We had a case conference on a 49-year old alcoholic woman. We decided that we need to work with her to mutually set goals rather than setting them for her." When transactions are made between nurses and clients, goals are attained. These nurses saw the need for negotiation in order for transaction to occur.

Role. "Miss W. has definite expectations of the nurses, eg., she expects help with her bath, etc., even though she doesn't need it. She needs to be reassured frequently. She accepts the role of the patient *very* well, as long as you behave the way she thinks nurses should behave." Role is a set of behaviors expected when occupying a position in a social system. This nurse understood that the patient's expectations of her role are not always the same as her own expectations.

"Mr. C. passed away recently and a newspaper article on his life revealed that he had not only been a teacher and a principal, but volunteered as a Boy Scout leader for 60 years. He took on the role of helping others explore life and learn about themselves. With a debilitating cardiovascular accident it must have felt quite different and frustrating to be the student, no longer the teacher." In this example the nurse understood that her patients have occupied other roles before assuming the patient role. This helped her to empathize with the losses they have incurred and helped her have a better feeling for who these individuals are as people.

Stress. "By giving adequate information to a patient before an upcoming procedure, I helped to reassure him and helped him understand and relax, thus reducing undue stress he might have had due to not knowing. Fear of the unknown puts a lot of stress on anyone." This nurse was able to recognize the deleterious effects of stress and did something about it before it became unbearable.

"Stress is coming in on the weekend to find you are short-staffed. Everyone on the floor is affected, including the patients." Nurses are expected to decrease stressors in the hospital for patients and families, yet all-too-few support systems are offered to reduce stressors for nurses.

Social System

A Social System is a configuration of relationships within a culture. Some examples are families, religious systems, educational systems, work systems, and peer groups. The following are some examples of nurses' comments about the concepts within the Social System.

Organization. "There are times when my personal goal of providing individualized nursing care to patients conflicts with the organization's unstated goals. It is a common practice in the hospital setting to routinize care, resembling an assembly-line approach. The end product is to treat patients like objects." In the role of the nurse, there is potential conflict, as one is responsible for functioning to achieve the goals of the organization and also the goals of professional nursing. The demands of an organization sometimes make it difficult to provide the kind of nursing care we would all like.

Decision Making. "Mrs. F. has an extensive wardrobe and is very conscious of her appearance. It is, therefore, very important for her self-image to be able to choose her wardrobe. It also gives her a sense of control and responsibility, since many of her activities of daily living are accomplished only with the nurse's assistance." The nurse realized that allowing a patient to make decisions helps her to gain control over the environment. Notice that other concepts were being used in conjunction with decision making.

"Mrs. M. has recently undergone a health experience that she perceives as threatening to her physical well-being and independence. As I entered her room to give her medication for 8 A.M., I suggested to her that she had a choice about having her morning care now, or if she preferred to rest longer in bed, we could arrange to help her after breakfast. The patient had slept poorly the night before. She chose to rest longer. In allowing her to make this decision, however small, I felt it gave her a sense of assuming responsibility for herself and thereby increased her self-esteem and independence. As an advocate for the patient, this allowed me to feel that I was caring for and nurturing the comfort and well-being of the patient."

Power. "K.S. controls her eating habits in an attempt to obtain bargaining power with her doctor, ie., she refuses to eat and drink until she is granted weekend passes. We nurses encourage and reinforce cooperation and try to direct her to use her power in a more positive and constructive manner, eg., 'if you eat and drink appropriately, you can get passes on the weekend.'" Exertion of power by one person is dependent on the acceptance of that power by another person. These nurses recognized that power is goal-directed and were able to assist a patient to use her power more appropriately to meet her goals.

Authority. "By our Certificate of Competence, we have the authority to use our knowledge to the best of our ability and to provide our patients with the best possible care and emotional support." This nurse realized that her special knowledge and skills are recognized and legally authorized by society.

"Some patients believe that we have authority over them based on our knowledge and expertise. Therefore, if they refuse to have some procedure done and a nurse informs them of the importance of the procedure, they will tend to comply. For example, a patient with a distended bladder didn't like to be catheterized. The nurse informed her of the importance of the catheterization and the patient complied, with excellent results." Before authority can be exercised in any situation, a person must be perceived as having legitimate authority. This nurse used the authority her role allows to influence a patient's decision.

Status. "A patient may assume that he has status on the unit by virtue of the fact that he has been on the unit for a longer period than others. This can often be noted at mealtimes in the dining room when he demands his 'special' table and place at that table." Recognition of the status needs of patients in hospitals is essential in giving effective nursing care. This nurse, in recognizing this patient's need for status within the patient group, allowed him to express this need.

"Mrs. S. is very conscious of status. When speaking to nurses, she always states 'the doctor' made some statement or other regarding her care." Nurses must be aware of individuals within an organization who will listen only to people they perceive to have status and use this awareness to achieve goals.

These may seem like simple, everyday examples, and indeed they are. What is fascinating, and sometimes poignant, is to realize how natural this is for the nurses. Although some of the terms were new for them, the ideas were not, so that talking about their practice in light of King's framework was not difficult.

While "Concept of the Month" was underway, we began highlighting King's concepts here and there whenever we had an opportunity. For example, in psychiatry, the nurses began using case conferences, and decided, as a feature of each conference, to incorporate the month's concept. During these discussions of patient care, other concepts naturally came into the discussion as well.

Sometimes the added insight provided by the unit manager helped nurses to link a particular concept to what they were doing. Soon, they were pointing out concepts to their colleagues, and then an important event occurred.

One night, at a point when the psychiatric unit had no manager, a patient known to our staff was admitted. Through a combination of circumstances, he became extremely violent, significantly damaging property, and threatening worse. To make a long story short, although they handled the situation well, the nurses were left feeling frustrated and powerless. In the discussion that followed, they discovered an avenue of recourse that had previously been unexplored. They glanced at a diagram of King's framework (conveniently posted everywhere) and the concepts in the *Social System* jumped out at them! POWER! AUTHORITY! DECISION MAKING! How could they use their power effectively to prevent this from happening again? They decided to use the event as a catalyst to discuss a number of concerns which had been brewing. They drafted a beautiful memo to the chief executive officer outlining their concerns. The memo intelligently communicated the urgency they were feeling without being inflammatory. As a result, a number of major changes, including a hospital-wide program for management of aggressive behavior, have occurred and the nurses felt empowered by having used the framework to stimulate their plan of action.

As mentioned previously, we highlighted concepts here and there whenever the opportunity arose. When nurses spoke about "problem" patients at the nurses' station, we, and the managers, helped nurses to see why a patient was behaving the way he or she was by examining the patient's perspective and seeing how particular concepts entered into the picture.

As an example, Mr. N., a frail, elderly and confused man, was given a Fisher-Price activity center—a toy with knobs and buttons and things to twiddle. The nurses were asked why he was playing with that thing, because from outward appearances it seemed to be demeaning for him. Jill, one of the nurses, explained that he wasn't playing with a toy, but was actually re-living his earlier *role* as an auto mechanic by tinkering with the gadgets. When the toy was taken away, he became fairly agitated and distressed. Jill had demonstrated how a consideration of the concept of role led to a creative approach to patient management.

CONCURRENT STRATEGIES

If a conceptual model is supposed to provide a framework for nursing, we thought that it should also drive the design of any new nursing programs. For example, when our diabetes education committee devised a new teaching program for patients, it was based on the systems and concepts of King. When the hospital recognized a need to educate staff about the effective and therapeutic management of aggressive behavior, it too was based on King's framework. It was the same with our Nursing Quality Assurance program. In this way, we have tried to thread King's systems and concepts into just about everything that happens in our department.

Our medical units base their nursing case conferences on the conceptual framework. The pediatric unit manual is also structured according to King's framework.

When new managers join our department, we set aside a half day in which to indoctrinate them. We have a casual discussion about King's Conceptual Framework and its history at Centenary Hospital. Our main purpose, though, is to help them to discover how the concepts can apply in *their own clinical area*. We want them to leave our session thinking that King created the conceptual framework for their own clinical area. When new staff nurses join our directorate, in addition to being exposed to King's concepts during the general nursing orientation, they receive an exercise book specific to their clinical area to help them practice applying the concepts.

Remember that 23-page nursing history and assessment record? At this point, each clinical area has revised the tool to suit its special needs. Some areas are just beginning a trial of their new form, while other areas are well into their final revision.

Some nursing units have recently piloted a tool designed by the Nursing Practice Committee. The tool categorizes North America Nursing Diagnosis Association nursing diagnoses according to the systems and concepts of King's Conceptual Framework. The hospital had decided to employ nursing diagnoses but was hesitant to have their use seen as a separate exercise from that of using a theory base to guide the nursing process. The nurses who used the tool experimentally found that they could see the connection between nursing diagnoses and the conceptual framework. We hope to begin using the tool to help launch the use of nursing diagnoses on a hospital-wide basis.

THE FUTURE

We anticipate that the work we have already done linking nursing diagnoses with King's Conceptual Framework will provide a foundation for future computerization. It is our hope that computer software designed from a nursing framework will be superior to what we have seen thus far in shopping for computer systems. Current computer systems for nursing that we have investigated fail to encompass the totality of the person and seem to add the nonphysical aspects of care as an afterthought.

We spoke earlier of the proposed College of Nurses of Ontario Standards. As we move to computerization, we hope to be able to incorporate these standards into the systems and concepts of our chosen framework. In this way, the legislative guidelines for our nursing practice can be read and understood in the context of our theoretical base. This would have the additional advantage of making our governing body's mandate more meaningful to our nursing department.

The idea of moving to adopt King's Theory of Goal Attainment intrigues us as a next step. Through our work to date, our nurses are gaining a solid foundation in the conceptual framework. As we move through the nursing process in our implementation, (and remember we have only been dealing with assessment and diagnosis to date), King's theory will provide direction for the evaluation phase. We could also then use the Theory of Goal Attainment to realize more measurable quality assurance outcomes.

We have not begun to run out of ideas yet. The process of applying theory to practice is just that—a process. As we go along, we are gaining new awareness of the potential that this particular framework gives us.

It has not been as easy as it may have sounded here. We have some units in our hospital which are experiencing difficulty understanding the usefulness of the framework for their clinical areas. They are now beginning to discover that implementing theory-based practice really isn't something "extra." It's part of what they do every day.

We, too, experienced times of waning enthusiasm and sometimes wondered if we were stepping backward and not forward. It was necessary to employ some morale-boosting strategies to inject new life once the novelty had begun to wear off. "Kingratulations" parties were held for no particular reason other than to celebrate the completion of all the concepts in any one system during that drawn-out Concept of the Month exercise. We were also fortunate to have King as our guest during the summer of 1988. This "Royal Visit," in which King made a walkabout tour of the nursing units and held a discussion with staff, did a great deal to excite everyone. To see that Imogene King is a real live nurse who could understand, sympathize with, and speak the same language as a staff nurse did more to boost morale than we could ever have hoped.

CONCLUSION

In conclusion, we would recommend that anyone considering implementing a conceptual framework or theory into practice at an agency should not be afraid to take the plunge. All it takes is some perseverance, flexibility, and a sense of humor. We believe that the serious nature of nursing theory is not diminished by occasional lightheartedness.

As professionals, we nurses must be prepared to articulate our discrete body of knowledge to ourselves, to other health care professionals, and to the public. We need to know what we are doing as nurses and why we are doing it. Only in this way can we validate our mandate as a profession. It sounds simple, but it has not been happening. In order to do this, we need to reflect on our practice and in order to pull it all together we need a framework. We have provided King's Conceptual Framework for our nurses and they have shown evidence of "pulling it all together" by identifying the theoretical basis of their own practice. The future is here.

REFERENCE

King, I. (1981). *Toward a theory for nursing: Systems, concepts, process*. New York: John Wiley & Sons.

Part 5

Martha Rogers' Theoretical Framework for Nursing

10

Space-Age Paradigm for New Frontiers in Nursing

Martha E. Rogers

In February 1957, Lee DeForest, father of modern electronics, stated: "To place a man in a multistage rocket and propel him into the controlling gravitational field of the moon . . . . will never occur regardless of all future scientific endeavors" and compared such proposals to the wildest dreams of Jules Verne (Friedman, 1989). This was just 12 years before the Apollo moon landing.

Manned voyages to Mars now seem likely by the year 2000, with a projected round trip of as little as two months (*Futurific*, Feb. 1990). Currently, 125 students from 26 countries are enrolled in the International Space University—an international, nonprofit, interdisciplinary institution designed to educate the world's future space professionals (Burke, 1989). Out of 2,500 applicants to the National Aeronautics and Space Administration (NASA) for admission to the Astronaut Corps in 1990, 106 made it to the interview stage—all expertly qualified in diverse scientific and technological fields. At the end of the process, 23 applicants were selected. Numbers of astronauts to be selected are increasing, but competition is sharp. Technical skill, enthusiasm, communication skills, and experience in areas outside one's own discipline are essential, but the sine qua non of being an astronaut is generally noted as the ability to be a team player (Triplett, 1990).

Increasing space travel capabilities are manifest in many countries. Establishment of moon villages, space towns, and Martian communities are near and presage a major emigration of "earthkind" in the not too distant future. Interplanetary and intergalactic communication with intelligent life beyond our present purview portends new meanings to citizenship in a space-encompassing world society. Interestingly enough, each dollar NASA spends for research and development generates $9.00 in private spending (*Futurific,* Feb. 1990).

A new oneness attends planet Earth's integration into the space world: a new synthesis in which spin-off from space exploration marks planet Earth's future.

Astronauts—precursors of "spacekind"—portend outward emigration by Homo sapiens and their transcendence by "Homo spatialis." This transcendence will be an evolutionary process, not an adaptive one. According to Robinson and White (1986), this process could take place in two generations of space living (about 50 years). Life support systems in reverse will then be needed for the earth-bound traveler from space. (There are those who are already predicting a shortage of Homo sapiens on planet Earth as emigration expands.) A cartoon in a recent issue of *Omni* depicts two Homo spatialis by the bedside of a very sick "Earthman." One "Spaceman" is saying to the other "If he lives he'll be nothing more than a Homo sapiens."

New world views abound. Synthesis and holism are predominant among these views. James Lovelock, in *The Ages of Gaia* (1988), proposes a scientific synthesis in harmony with the Greek conception of the Earth as a living whole, as Gaia. Buckminster Fuller (1981) argues firmly for Earth as a spaceship. Leslie Kenton, writing in the *Noetic Sciences Bulletin* (1990), emphasizes the fallacy of depending on well-meaning actions and good intentions while we continue to operate with a paradigm that views reality as fragmented. Holistic world views are being studied by such persons as David Bohm, Fritz Capra, Rupert Sheldrake and, Rene Weber—both as individuals and in groups. My own work focuses on developing a holistic world view by proposing a science of unitary, irreducible beings that is coordinate with a world view that includes outer space.

Noninvasive therapeutic modalities are increasingly emphasized by a range of health care workers. New modalities will emerge out of evolution toward spacekind, which will spark more effective modalities for earthkind. A holistically oriented space-age paradigm is the substance of nursing's science of unitary, irreducible human beings.

Traditional world views are increasingly untenable and fail to explain contemporary events. Today's health care system is dangerously deficient and cannot be cured simply by adding more dollars or by other simplistic proposals. Toxic terrorists abound. Remember the two grapes from Chile and the Alar apples from Washington state. Colman McCarthy in an Editorial in *The Washington Post* last year wrote, "Dairy cows are shot through with so many drugs that milk ought to be sold as a prescription-only product." *Science News* in its September 23, 1989, issue notes "Green House warming is being recognized as a terrorist threat—not a scientific reality." The *Baltimore Sun* recently headlined a wire-service story thus: "Cow gas blamed for global warming." Another report based on ten years of weather satellite data shows no evidence of global warming from the greenhouse effect (*Arizona Republic,* March 1990). The debate goes on.

AIDS doesn't kill everyone who gets the virus. Infectious diseases are not new to this planet. Hope, attitude, mood, and laughter are reported to be as effective in strengthening the autoimmune system as drugs and vaccines. Today's major health problem is nosophobia: a morbid dread of disease.

Denial of human freedom to select medical care other than allopathic has helped spawn the Coalition for Alternatives in Nutrition and Health Care, a group that is promoting a health care rights amendment which would prohibit Congress from making any law restricting individuals' rights to choose and practice the type of health care they want.

As nurses move into the mainstream of a growing entrepreneurial society, subtle harassment and euphemisms are not unknown deterrents to nurses and are further aggravated by nurses who support anti-educationism in nursing and dependency on others. Failure to value differences between nurses and other health care personnel adds to the problem.

Accelerating change, an unpredictable future, and mushrooming social and ethical issues threaten the status-quoers. James Madison, in a speech given June 16, 1788, made this statement:

> I believe there are more instances of the abridgement of the freedom of the people by gradual and silent encroachments of those in power than by violent and sudden usurpation.

A humorous note seems fitting here:

> What with the threat of nuclear war, acid rain, crime in the streets, and AIDS—sometimes it seems as if it hardly pays to give up smoking.

Nursing is inseparable from the new world view and the process of change. Holistic trends are on the way to becoming a massive torrent. A new vision of a world encompassing far more than planet Earth is in the making. The science of nursing emerges out of a space-age world view. The evidence of diversifying wholeness is substantial. For instance the pace of evolution from clans to tribes to city-states to nation-states to one planet is accelerating.

THE SCIENCE OF NURSING

My discussion of nursing begins with the premise that nursing is a learned profession: a science and an art. A science is an organized body of abstract knowledge. The art involved in nursing is the creative use of science for human betterment. As a science, nursing generates many theories.

The uniqueness of nursing, as in other sciences, is identified in the phenomena of concern. Nursing is the study of unitary, irreducible human beings and their respective environments. As a science, the term "nursing" is a noun signifying an organized body of abstract knowledge. Theories of nursing derive from this abstract system of knowledge. The science of unitary human beings is rooted in a new world view coordinate with today's knowledge. The science of nursing is a synthesis of facts and ideas; it is a new product.

Many fields emerge out of new world views, holistic in focus. Fields differ according to the phenomena of concern. The following attributes are some of those included in the holistic world view presented here.

- *Energy Fields:* The fundamental unit of the living and the nonliving. Field is a unifying concept. Energy signifies the dynamic nature of the field. Fields are infinite and continuously open.
- *Pattern:* The distinguishing characteristic of an energy field perceived as a single wave.
- *Multidimensional:* A nonlinear domain without spatial or temporal attributes.

The above terms represent definitions of a specificity within the science of nursing. General language definitions are relevant unless a term is defined with specificity. Two further terms of significance in this world view are defined as follows:

- *Unitary Person:* An irreducible, multidimensional energy field identified by pattern and manifesting characteristics that are specific to the whole and cannot be predicted from knowledge of the parts.
- *Environment:* An irreducible multidimensional energy field identified by pattern and integral with a given human field.

People *are* energy fields. They do not have them. Continuous change emerges out of nonequilibrium and exhibits punctualism not gradualism. Change is accelerating. Chaos theory is transforming the way we think the world is (Crum, 1989; Peterson, 1989; Percival, 1989; Stewart, 1989).

Principles of Homeodynamics

Principles of Homeodynamics derive from the abstract system and postulate the nature of change. The principles are listed as follows.

- *Principle of Resonancy:* The continuous change from lower to higher frequency wave patterns in human and environmental fields.
- *Principle of Helicy:* The continuous innovative, unpredictable, increasing diversity of human and environmental field patterns.
- *Principle of Integrality:* The continuous mutual human field and environmental field process.

Manifestations of field pattern assist in relating the abstract to the everyday world.

Manifestations of Field Patterning in Unitary Human Beings

The evolution of unitary human beings is a dynamic, irreducible, nonlinear process characterized by increasing diversity of energy field patterning. Manifestations of patterning emerge out of the mutual human/environmental field process and are continuously changing. Pattern is an abstraction that reveals itself through its manifestations.

The nature of unitary field patterning is unpredictable and creative. Change is relative and increasingly diverse. Some manifestations of relative diversity in field patterning are noted below.

Individuals experience lesser diversity and greater diversity, longer rhythms, shorter rhythms, and rhythms that seem continuous. Individuals experience motion as slower, faster, and continuous. Individuals experience time as slower, faster, or unmoving. Individuals are sometimes pragmatic, sometimes imaginative, and sometimes visionary. Individuals experience periods of longer sleeping, longer waking, and periods of being beyond waking.

NURSING EDUCATION AND PRACTICE

The world view and abstract system I present encompass earthkind and spacekind. Manifestations of change are holistic, continuous, and manifestations of pattern emerging out of the human and environmental field process. Homo spatialis is a product of evolution

—a new species transcending Homo sapiens. It should be noted that changes that occur in Homo sapiens in space need not be labeled pathology. In fact, one would properly perceive such changes as manifestations of the human and environmental field process. This world view and this abstract system represent a new reality. The new reality encompasses new ways of thinking, new questions, new interpretations—and requires consistency with the system if one is to study it. Stephen Jay Gould wrote in the *Natural History Journal* a comment of relevance here, "Facts do not speak for themselves. They are read in the light of theory." Research and investigation in the science of unitary human beings is on-going (Malinski, 1986; Barrett, 1990; Sarter, 1990).

The study of nursing as a science is the study of the phenomena central to nursing; unitary, irreducible human beings and their environments. It is *not* the study of other fields or theories deriving from other fields. A sociological theory is just that, no matter who studies it. Such a theory may be very good and the investigator may make a significant contribution to sociology. The study of nurses and what they do is not the study of nursing anymore than the study of biologists and what they do is the study of biology.

The education of nurses, whether technical, professional, or advanced, is properly rooted in a sound general education appropriate to the level of preparation sought. Everyone needs to include extraterrestrial content in their learning.

Central to the education of nurses must be study of the science of unitary human beings. Further, we must commit ourselves to a lifetime of learning. The nature of the practice of nursing (the use of knowledge for human betterment) is rooted in what one knows and in the imagination, creativity, compassion, and skill one uses. Nurses focus on health promotion. In the educational process we do not need to teach students how to do everything. Rather we need to teach them how to figure out how to do everything.

Health services are community based. Services such as hospitals, nursing homes, and the like supplement the base. There is a great need among all health care workers to develop mutual respect for differences.

Noninvasive modalities mark the future of nursing practice on this planet and in outer space. Therapeutic touch, imagery, meditation, relaxation, and the like will increase. Diversifying wholeness emphasizes the growing need for more individualization of services. Nonrepeating rhythmicities in sound, color, taste, fragrance, and the like have undreamed of potentials. Caring is a practice modality getting much attention from nurses, but caring does not identify nurses any more than workers in any other field. Almost everyone is capable of caring. The nature of caring in a given field depends on the body of scientific knowledge specific to that field. Humor, laughter, mood, and attitude have been found to be significant in health promotion and maintenance.

As a holistic reality revolutionizes our thinking and as space exploration and space living provide spin-off from space that can be helpful on planet Earth, nursing will change, as will other fields. We are on the threshold of a fantastic and unimagined future. Our potential for human service is greater than it has ever been. On with it!

REFERENCES

Barrett, E. (1990). *Visions of Rogers' science-based nursing.* New York: National League for Nursing.

Burke, J. T. (1989). ISU tunes in on voyager watch. *The planetary report, IX*(6), 4.

Cow gas blamed. (1990, March). *Arizona Republic,* p. A6.

Crum, R. (1989, fall). Why Johnny kills. *New York University Magazine, 4*(2), 34.

Each dollar NASA spends. (1990, February). *Futurific, 14*(2), 37.

Friedman, S. T. (1989, February). Who believes in UFO's? *International UFO Reporter, 14*(1), 6-10.

Fuller, R. B. (1981). Critical Path. New York: St. Martin's Press.

Gould, S. J. (1977, February). This view of life. *Natural History, 52,* 20-24.

Kenton, L. (1990, spring). Member forum. *Noetic Sciences Bulletin, V*(1), 6.

Lovelock, J. (1988). *The ages of Gaia.* New York: W.W. Norton & Co.

Malinski, V. (1986). *Explorations of Martha Rogers' science of unitary human beings.* Norwalk, CT: Appleton-Century-Crofts.

Manned voyages to Mars. (1990, February). *Futurific, 14*(2), 37.

Percival, I. (1989, October). Chaos: A science for the real world. *New Scientist, 123,* 42–47.

Peterson, I. (1989, July). Digging into sand. *Science News, 136,* 40.

Robinson, G., & White, H. (1986). *Envoys of mankind.* Washington: Smithsonian Institution Press.

Sarter, B. (1988). *The stream of becoming: A study of Martha Rogers' theory.* New York: National League for Nursing.

Stewart, I. (1989). *Does God play dice?: The mathematics of chaos.* Cambridge, MA: Brasil Blackwell, Inc.

Triplett, W. (1990, April/May). The class of 1990. *Air & Space, 5*(1), 73–77.

11

Practical Application of Rogers' Theoretical Framework for Nursing

Linda Joseph

Martha Rogers' framework for nursing, introduced in her book, *An Introduction to the Theoretical Basis of Nursing,* is an inspiration and a challenge. This chapter provides an overview of the Rogerian framework and how it's application guides and enriches nursing practice.

ROGERS' VIEW: A WORLD VIEW FOR NURSING

In her book, Rogers clearly articulates what is for many nurses an unspoken, deep inner knowing of what nursing is. She provides a context for the meaning of nursing and a description of the world in which we nurse. What Rogers gives us is a world view. It is a holistic world view that resolves the disparity nurses feel between the mechanistic, reductionist viewpoint predominant in medical model systems and the whole human beings that are the focus of nursing interactions.

Basic Postulates of the Rogerian Framework

Within a holistic world view, the Rogerian framework takes form as a "Science of Unitary Human Beings" that is based on the following postulates.

- *The person is a unified whole.* We cannot study the biology, sociology, psychology, and so forth of a human being and know the person as a whole. A human being is multidimensional, and is *greater than* and *different from* the sum of his or her parts. A whole human being cannot be known through reduction to systems, organs, and cells.
- *The person is characterized as a human energy field.* This concept unifies the multiple dimensions of the person's wholeness and names this unity the human energy field.
- *The unified human energy field is an open system, constantly exchanging matter and energy with the environment, which is itself a greater energy field that extends to infinity.* The whole of each human energy field interacts with the whole of its environment in a dynamic, ongoing energy exchange that is life. We observe and live these exchanges every day personally and in our nursing practices. Some simple examples of energy exchanges are eating, speaking, breathing, and emoting. Energy exchanges are simultaneous processes of change and creation unique to each person and his or her environmental field; they are *not* cause and effect relationships.
- *The identity and integrity of the human energy field is maintained through patterning and organization.* The order of life is maintained through constant change. Patterns are expressed in rhythmical relationships within each human energy field and between the human and environmental energy fields. We see evidence of this in physiological patterns such as those involved in sleeping-waking, temperature, and hormonal cycles. Patterns may also be viewed in tendencies of thought and spirituality, such as values, attitudes, and beliefs that are unique to each human energy field. In the environmental field of each person's world, we see patterns and rhythms of energy exchange such as work, recreation, and social alliances.

HOMEOSTASIS IS OUT; HOMEODYNAMICS ARE IN

In a world view where person and environment are in a constant, dynamic, simultaneous process of change, the concept of homeostasis is obsolete. Rogers' principles of homeodynamics add further detail to the Rogerian conceptual system of nursing and the life process. According to Malinsky (1986), the principles of homeodynamics, "describe the nature and direction of change manifested by unitary human beings in mutual process with the environment." The dynamic, rhythmical process of energy exchange between humans and their respective environments is in the direction of greater diversity, complexity, creation, innovation, and fulfillment of potential. Individual ability to know oneself and one's world allows one to reflect, choose, and engage consciously in the process of life. This is the realm of nursing's focus.

NURSING: THE ROGERIAN WAY

Rogers (1970) states, "The phenomenon central to nursing . . . is the life process in man." The health of a human energy field is simply what is true about that person's interaction between self and the environment in that moment. Our professional role as nurses is to serve people in this process. We are challenged to look at patients, friends, strangers, and ourselves in this context and redefine our nursing activities accordingly.

How can nurses facilitate clients in their processes of life and health within this framework? To explore this most fully, I would like to share how the Rogerian framework may be applied to the design and implementation of a health care program and how it may be applied through a specific nursing modality—Therapeutic Touch.

THE ROGERIAN FRAMEWORK: A BLUEPRINT FOR HEALTH CARE

I had the wonderful opportunity to develop and coordinate an inpatient/outpatient, interdisciplinary program for the management of chronic pain within an acute care hospital setting. In preparation for this undertaking, a team of professionals versed in the healing arts as well as health sciences—the traditional and nontraditional approaches within their disciplines—was gathered. An appreciation for the energetic wholeness of human beings was a prerequisite for hire. In round table discussions this team conceived the philosophy, conceptual framework, and mission of the program—using the Rogerian framework as the guiding model for clinical practice.

Interdisciplinary Applications of the Rogerian Framework

While the unitary human being is the unique focus of professional nursing, I believe the world view described by Rogers is appropriate as a framework for the practice of any human-science discipline. It was recognized by our team that a person experiencing chronic illness, such as chronic pain, is experiencing energetic disruption physically, mentally, emotionally, spiritually, socially, vocationally, and so on. While it is the role of the nurse to address the health situation of the person as a unified whole and facilitate that person's process holistically, the team representatives of other disciplines addressed specific dimensions of this process. For example, the team psychologist primarily addressed the psycho-emotional and spiritual dimensions and the rehabilitation counselor addressed the vocational aspects.

The intention of the team was to create a *team energy field* that would become the clients' environments and would allow them to reflect on and explore their situations; recognize and choose options; and create greater harmony, vitality, and well-being for themselves. Clients were not reduced to parts that we could do things to; rather, we constantly referenced their energetic wholeness.

Patterning: The Choreography of Wellness

The focus of the health care team was identification of the patterns of each person-environment and facilitation of a repatterning process, as appropriate. For example, the physical therapist explored posture and movement patterns and assisted clients in repatterning for greater safety, strength, flexibility, and stamina. The psychologist explored patterns of communication and of repression of unresolved emotional issues. By assisting clients in addressing these areas, energy was freed for more effective healing and management of the pain problem. The vocational rehabilitation counselor addressed the clients' abilities and unique needs in interacting with their work environments in order to achieve an appropriate occupational match. The physician, also using the holistic model, addressed drug taking and worked with clients to repattern drug-taking behaviors. He also worked with clients to reconcile any confusion they might be having in experiencing the holistic, nonmedical model in this health care setting.

INTEGRATING THE ROGERIAN MODEL INTO NURSING CARE

The nurse, true to the Rogerian framework for nursing, coordinated the dynamics of the client as a total person in this all-encompassing repatterning process. In an orientational session, nurses introduced clients to the holistic world view used by the professionals in the program. Nurses engaged in educational processes, interpersonal communication, and various traditional and nontraditional nursing approaches to facilitate the clients' overall experience.

While every nurse may not have the opportunity to create a health care program from scratch, we all choose the way we interact with clients in our varied practices. Every nurse has the opportunity to reflect upon his or her world view and how it relates to the care given. To begin to bring the Rogerian framework into practical application, this is all that is necessary. To get started, you may wish to do a little retrospective study each day that you work. Take a few moments to reflect on just one client, the energetic patterns you observed between that human energy field and his or her environment and the patterns that you as a caregiving human energy field engaged in with this client. Gradually, this process of reflection shifts from being retrospective to being something that you do as you interact with your clients. Very quickly you begin to have greater insight into clients, their worlds, their health situations, and ways that you can serve them in this process.

THERAPEUTIC TOUCH: A ROGERIAN NURSING MODALITY

Moving on now to a specific nursing modality as an application of the Rogerian framework, I will present the way the nurses in this same pain management center used Therapeutic Touch (TT) with clients. Therapeutic Touch is a technique developed at New York University by Dr. Dolores Krieger, a professor of nursing. It is grounded in the world view and theoretical framework for nursing described by Rogers. In the Pain Management Center, beginning with an educational class entitled "Personal Energy Management," clients were introduced to the idea and experience of themselves as human energy fields within an energetic environment. They were assisted in exploring the unique nature, patterns, and relationships of their energy exchanges with the environment. This awareness allowed them to contemplate and move toward actualizing new patterns of energy exchange that better served them. For example, clients completed an energy assessment tool in which they listed those life experiences that stimulate or enhance their energy and those that deplete it, in the realms of body, mind, and spirit. These delineations were not meant to fragment or reduce clients to parts, rather, to help them to identify their multidimensional involvement with their environments. Identifying their own patterns of energy depletion and replenishment empowered clients to make decisions to repattern their energy exchanges in greater alignment with what they desired for themselves.

Following this class, clients were seen on an individual basis for four to 12 TT sessions. While these sessions began with TT in the traditional sense of the practice, we went on to assist clients in developing their own energy strategies for well-being. The process of TT reflects the Rogerian framework and how it was of benefit to the clients we served.

Therapeutic Touch: an Overview

Dolores Krieger (1979) described three prerequisites to the effective practice of TT. The first is examining our *motivation,* that is, we must explore our motivation in choosing nursing, choosing to engage in interaction with other human energy fields in environments and ways designed to facilitate them in their health process. To address this prerequisite, apply a variation of the self-study exercise recommended earlier. Each day you work, reflect on one client you cared for and explore what your motivation was in your interactions with this client.

At times, our motivations are more selfless; we are clearly present to support the clients in their processes and attend fully to this. At other times we are more selfish, not in a judgmental sense, but it is just the way of the world that at times our own needs and concerns are foremost in our minds. When this is the case, our full energies may not be available to the clients we serve. Knowing this assists us to best meet our clients' needs despite the various demands on our attention and energy.

Another prerequisite noted by Krieger is *centering.* Centering is the act of quieting and focusing, stepping outside of daily concerns and being as present as possible to the situation at hand. Centering is cultivated through a discipline of practicing any technique which assists in arriving at that still, yet strong and focused place within. Examples of some practices that help people gain skill in centering are relaxation or breathing exercises, biofeedback, meditation, prayer, running, music, and imagery. By daily practice of any method that enhances access of a centered state, greater and greater ability to become centered by choice at any time is gained. In the centered state, we are more sensitive to the energetic realms of our clients.

Yet another prerequisite is *intentionality.* It is conscious intention that focuses our energy and the ways we exchange energy in nursing practice. When a nurse enters a client's room to administer a medication, is the intention to get in and out as quickly as possible, get on to other clients, and get out of work on time to pick up the kids? This is a valid intention that may be underlying all of our actions at work one day. Yet, how much more effective is a nurse-client interaction if before entering the client's room the nurse can center and consciously hold the intention that the medication take effect quickly and gently and produce maximal comfort, minimal side effects, and maximal therapeutic results?

Simply engaging in a self-study of motivation and intention, augmented by a commitment to develop skill in centering, can enrich each nurse's practice tremendously. Begin today to enhance your nursing career by exploring your relationship to these prerequisites.

THE THERAPEUTIC TOUCH EXPERIENCE

The presentation of TT as a practice skill is beyond the scope of this chapter. The following is a simplified overview of TT, how it was used in clinical practice at the Pain Management Center, and how it relates to the Rogerian framework.

In the study of TT, people are viewed as human energy fields. Caregivers learn to tune in to the latent capacity we all have to sense the human energy field, which includes and extends outwardly from the physical body. By placing your hands opposite one another and repeatedly moving them together until they are almost touching and then moving them apart, as though you were playing an invisible accordion, you may begin to feel subtle sensations in your palms or fingertips. Perhaps you feel a sensation of heat, or tingling; perhaps pressure as you move your hands together, or a drawing sensation as you gently move them apart. What you are feeling is your own energy field through the tactile ability of your hands to sense the human energy field.

Using our hands, we can sense the character of another's energy field and engage in an energy exchange with that person to facilitate his or her energetic status toward greater vitality, harmony, balance, and well-being. This is done by centering so as to attend to the subtleties of the energetic field, and then moving the hands through the field of the other person, approximately 3–5" from his or her body, in order to detect any differences from one area of the field to another. Differences represent potential energetic disturbances in the human energy field. Once these areas are identified, the caregiver can engage in an energy exchange with the client, again, using his or her hands as the focus for therapeutic intent. This time, the intention is to clear and mobilize the field of the client and make energy available to the client's field, thereby harmonizing his or her energetic exchange with the environment.

INTEGRATING THERAPEUTIC TOUCH INTO NURSING PRACTICE: AN EXAMPLE

At the Pain Management Center, TT was offered to each client after he or she attended a "Personal Energy Management" class in which the energetic perspective was explained. As previously mentioned, it was the intention not to "do things to" clients, but rather, to assist them in gaining skills they could use themselves. This raised a challenge to design an approach in which TT could be offered in this light.

Personal Energy Management: Self Health Through Therapeutic Touch

To begin, clients were interviewed regarding their perception of their own energy status. Were their energy levels high or low; focused or agitated and scattered. Did they feel energetically vulnerable to situations in their environment and out of control? Did their energies support them physically, mentally, and spiritually as they desired? Using TT in the traditional way, an assessment and treatment was done. In subsequent sessions, new information was gathered and as early as clients were willing and able to assume responsibility, they were taught to use energy self-help exercises to energetically support themselves. These might include, for example, breathing techniques, self-massage, or use of music or imagery—all powered by focused therapeutic energetic intentions. All clients are unique; their issues of energy exchange with the environment are unique; and the personal energy plan created with each client was, therefore, also unique. Each client was assisted by all members of the team to integrate and apply self-help skills into daily life.

As a component of the program, TT sessions were charged as nursing visits and documented in the medical record. Since the institution used nursing diagnosis, the client situation was defined as "Alterations in Energy Balance" and was described in the notes. Notes included what the client stated about his or her energy status, what we perceived in the energy assessment, what took place during the treatment and/or application of self-help techniques, and the client's response in energetic terms.

THERAPEUTIC TOUCH AND THE ROGERIAN FRAMEWORK

In TT, clients are addressed as human energy fields. Nurses engage in a process of exploring with clients the nature of their energetic exchange with the environment. Through TT, clients are assisted in creating innovative ways to promote their energetic well-being and move in the direction of their choice, toward actualizing their potential. While you cannot read this chapter and expect to engage in the practice of TT, you may begin today to view your clients as unified, holistic beings. You can take the perspective of exploring with them the nature and quality of their energetic exchanges with their environments. You can support them in taking the opportunity their health situation has given them to engage with you in the process of patterning their energies moment by moment, interaction by interaction in ways that serve them. Further, if you are inspired and challenged by Rogers' framework for nursing, you can direct your energy to reading, studying, and attending other seminars and conferences that will support you in your knowledge and practice of the Rogerian framework.

REFERENCES

Borelli, M. D., & Heidt, P. (1981). *Therapeutic Touch: A book of readings*. New York: Springer.

Jurgens, A., Meehan, T. C., & Wilson, H. L. (1987). Therapeutic Touch as a nursing intervention. *Holistic Nursing Practice, 2*(1), 1–13.

Krieger, D. (1979). *The Therapeutic Touch: How to use your hands to help or to heal.* Englewood Cliffs, N.J.: Prentice-Hall.

Krieger, D. (1981). *Foundations for holistic health nursing practices: The renaissance nurse.* Philadelphia: J.B. Lippincott.

Krieger, D. (1988). *Living the Therapeutic Touch: Healing as a lifestyle.* New York: Dodd, Mead & Co.

Macrae, J. (1987). *Therapeutic Touch: A practical guide.* New York: Alfred A. Knopf.

Malinsky, V. (1986). *Explorations on Martha Rogers' science of unitary human beings.* Norwalk, CT: Appleton-Century-Crofts.

Newman, M. A. (1986). *Health as expanding consciousness.* St. Louis: C.V. Mosby.

Rogers, M. E. (1970). *An introduction to the theoretical basis of nursing.* Philadelphia: F.A. Davis.

Quinn, J. (1988). Building a body of knowledge: Research on Therapeutic Touch, 1974-1986. *Journal of Holistic Nursing, 6*(1), 37-45.

Sarter, B. (1987). Evolutionary idealism: A philosophical foundation for holistic nursing theory. *Advances in Nursing Science, 9*(2), 1-9.

Sarter, B. (1988). *The stream of becoming: A study of Martha Rogers' theory.* New York: National League for Nursing.

Part 6

Newman's Theory of Health

12

Shifting to Higher Consciousness

Margaret A. Newman

We are living in a very interesting time. Some would call it a new age, but it is no longer so new anymore. We are living in a time of breaking down barriers, of breaking down hierarchical structures, of crossing over boundaries. We are moving into a time of increasing cooperation between people, people who have different ideas. We are moving into a time of mutuality and of caring and, I would say, a time of higher consciousness and greater freedom of choice all around the world.

This shift is taking place in nursing as well. While on leave from the University of Minnesota, I studied the nursing case manager model of practice at Carondelet St. Mary's Health Center in Tucson, Arizona. I spent three months getting to know the nurse case managers and learning about their practice. The nurse case managers relate to clients on a continuing basis wherever the client may be: in the hospital, in the home, in the clinic, in the nursing home, and if necessary, in the hospital again. This freedom to follow the client wherever the client needs to be is a dimension of practice that has been long needed (Newman, 1975). A professional is not bound by space or time and is free to move across institutional boundaries (Newman, 1990a).

The nurse case managers function as a group, as a nursing network; decisions affecting their practice are made by the group. In this way, the hospital walls are no longer a barrier to the relationship between nurse and client, and the structure of the nurses' practice is nonhierarchical.

The nurse case managers emphasized that the most meaningful part of their practice was the relationship formed with the client. It was the nature of this relationship that was most important. The relationship was difficult for the case managers to define, but they said it was something akin to friendship. It was characterized by mutuality. Certainly caring was a part of this relationship. The mutuality of the relationship was such that both the client and the nurse experienced personal transformation, or as I later realized, the expansion of consciousness. A part of the practice was letting go of the "professional" agenda and getting in touch with the evolving pattern of the client, getting in touch with the person as a whole, and following their individual pathway.

When the nurse case managers talked about their relationships with other health care professionals, they depicted a cooperative alliance formed to serve the client. Serving the client was the key. If they lost sight of that mission, turf issues could arise.

Actually, the term "case management" was a misnomer. They were not managing a case or managing a client. They were interacting in a mutual, cooperative partnership with the client. The word used most often to describe what they did was *facilitating* the choices faced by the client. One nurse could not even go so far as to use the word facilitating because it, too, depicted to her a less than mutual process.

As I analyzed the data from my interviews with the nurse case managers, it seemed to me that their practice embodied the theory I have been talking about for the past 12 years. Sometimes I think of my theory strictly in terms of health (as expanding consciousness), but students point out to me that I have not been talking solely about health: I have been talking about the relationship that exists between nurse and client and the mutuality that occurs in the process of assisting clients in making and implementing their choices. As I reported my analysis to the case managers at St. Mary's, I suddenly saw their practice as the explication of my theory. They had not set out to apply my theory. They were practicing nursing as they saw it. Yet there was congruence between my theory and their practice.

This experience helped me understand my theory a little better. It is not something that one imposes on the situation. (Previously we were taught that theory is something separate that we test and test and test until we are sure we have got it right, and then we apply it.) One does not "lay it on." It seems to me that my theory is an *explication* of the experience of many nurses. This is what I hear when nurses call me and tell me that what I have written in my book (Newman, 1986) meant a lot to them because it expressed what they have been experiencing, but have not been able to put into words.

A prior step of my recent realizations about the theory is described in a recent article on the theory as praxis (Newman, 1990b). I now see the theory, the research, and the practice as one process—not separate entities. This is part of the shift in paradigm.

I am using the word "paradigm" simply to mean a world view. The world view of health for most of us, based on our education and careers, has been health as the absence of disease. Probably many of you will reject that notion and say, no, that is not what we are concerned with; we are concerned with wellness. The illness-wellness continuum, however, is part of the world view of health as the absence of disease because as one moves toward the wellness end of the continuum, or as we try to move clients toward the wellness end of the continuum, we are talking about moving the client away from disease by either preventing the disease or promoting behaviors that we think will promote health. The vast majority of reported nursing research supports this assertion (Newman, in press).

I am talking about a different way of viewing health, a paradigm shift. I am talking about a view that encompasses disease as a meaningful aspect of health.

It has helped me, in understanding this paradigm shift, to think about the Copernican shift. In the days of Copernicus, everyone thought the earth was the center of the universe and the sun and the other planets revolved around the earth. Copernicus said, on the basis of his calculations, that's not the way it is. The sun is the center of the universe, and the earth and all the other planets revolve around the sun. Aha! They were looking at the same things, but seeing them differently. At first it is hard to make the shift because one is so accustomed to the old way of seeing things. From a limited perspective, the sun comes up and the sun goes down, and it looks like it is revolving around the earth. When one really grasps the reality of the alternate view, however, one cannot go back to viewing it the other way.

The paradigm shift in nursing began when Martha Rogers (1970) asked what is the center of nursing's purpose and began to describe the living system differently than it had been described before. She described the human being as a unitary system that is open and in interaction with the environment—with no real boundaries. She described it in terms of pattern. Pattern as an identification of the wholeness of the person is basic to the theory of health as expanding consciousness. It is not the substance of our bodies that identifies the person; it is the pattern that identifies the person: the pattern of the way one moves, or the way one talks, the pattern that can be identified across space and time. The pattern is what identifies us.

Another assumption of this paradigm is that the pattern is evolving unidirectionally. From my standpoint, and that of a number of contemporary scholars (Bentov, 1978; Moss, 1981; Watson, 1989; Wilber, 1979), that direction is toward higher consciousness.

If you can accept these two assumptions, then you can begin to think of disease as a manifestation of expanding consciousness. If you accept that pattern is a manifestation of the person, and that the process of life moves in the direction of increasing complexity, diversity, and higher consciousness, then when something appears or becomes manifest, it follows that it is a manifestation of the evolving pattern; it is not something separate to be gotten rid of or squelched, but something to be regarded as a clue to the underlying pattern.

Early in the development of the theory of health as a state of expanding consciousness, the emphasis of my activities in theory development and research was on movement, time, and consciousness. My explicit views on health did not take form until I was preparing for the 1978 conference on nursing theory in New York. I realized I was really talking about a different way of viewing health, and I found it important to identify my assumptions.

The first assumption was that health encompasses disease as a meaningful aspect of health, as a manifestation of the underlying pattern of person-environment interaction. Even if the disease is eradicated, it does not change the underlying pattern. Back in 1978, this assumption felt right and had limited support from the field of biological rhythms and from the work of Bahnson and Bahnson (1966) on cancer. This assumption was on even firmer ground when a couple of years later, David Bohm (1980) published his book on wholeness and the implicate order. His theory of implicate order seemed to me to support the idea of disease as a manifestation of pattern. The implicate order referred to the unseen, underlying pattern and was considered to be of primary importance. Bohm explained that from time to time the explication of the unseen pattern comes forth in things that we can see, feel, hear, and touch, and because these manifestations are so much more real to us than the unseen pattern, we think of them as primary, but in reality they are secondary. The explication arises out of and disappears into the implicate order, like waves that appear on the surface of the ocean and then disappear. Bohm's theory of implicate order is consistent with the view that the disease pattern or any other explicating pattern of the system arose out of the underlying, unseen pattern.

It is hard to switch paradigms. It was not until many years after I was introduced to these ideas that they took hold for me, that I really began to grasp this new way of viewing health.

One experience that helped me look at health differently related to a friend who had hyperthyroidism. She had all of the typical symptoms of a full-blown case of hyperthyroidism and had been under the supervision of an endocrinologist for about a year, when he concluded that the medical treatment was ineffective and that she would need surgery. Before she made the decision to go ahead with surgery, she went to see Dora Kunz (Karagulla & Kunz, 1989), a clairvoyant who was able to visualize auras. She told me later that Kunz had indicated that her energy was going in every direction, but in a somewhat diminished intensity, probably related to the drugs she was on to suppress the thyroid. Kunz said that she knew she could not recommend to my friend that she conserve her energy or decrease the channels of her energy, because that represented her way of life. What she did recommend was that my friend make sure she took in enough energy to maintain her way of life.

Well, sure enough my friend was expending her energy in many directions. She was the oldest of nine children, who, along with her parents, called on her for assistance and advice. She was a member of a community of nuns who frequently visited her on their way to other places. She carried an exceptionally heavy teaching load. She could never say "no" to a request to chair or serve on various committees. She was a faithful friend to many and went out of her way to plan parties and perform other favors for her friends. You get the picture. Her energy was going in every direction, and at the same time, her busy schedule precluded her getting much sleep or having time to eat properly.

The disease was a manifestation of her pattern. She got some insight into her pattern, began to pace herself differently, and the symptoms disappeared. I do not want to imply that just changing the energy balance, in terms of the intake and output of energy, did the trick. That would be an instrumental approach, with a limited effect. The important factor was the *insight* she gained regarding her pattern. She got in sync with her pattern and allowed the transformation to take place. What Kunz did was to help my friend see her pattern and help her *facilitate* it rather than try to squelch it. The old way of looking at things would be to try to eliminate the activity of the thyroid by surgery or drugs as though it were separate from the life process of which it is a part. In retrospect, one might say the thyroid was trying to keep up with her, not the other way around.

This was an important insight for me. Rogers (1970) had said that health and illness are simply expressions of the life process, one no more important than the other. It is hard for those of us who have been educated in the medical paradigm to see that one is no more important than the other. We have viewed them as polarized concepts; we have tried to promote health and avoid illness. Yet if you begin to see the unfolding pattern as a unitary process (an important dimension in the paradigm shift), the disease is not separate from health.

Another thing that was helpful in understanding this phenomenon as a unitary process was the study of biological rhythms. This is illustrated in the rhythms of body temperature. There are times when body temperature is above "normal" and times when it is below "normal." The temperature fluctuates in a circadian pattern. The meaning of the temperature lies in the overall pattern, which is unitary. There are times when it is important for the temperature to reach an extreme state in order to shift the system over into another way of functioning. There is a theoretical position within the study of biological rhythms that asserts that at times rhythms become increasingly disorganized until the system is shocked into another level of organization. The disorder and order, the disorganization and organization, the disharmony and harmony are all part of this rhythmic process.

Ilya Prigogine, a chemist and winner of the Nobel Prize for his theory of dissipative structures, described this when he wrote that he sees the organism or living system as functioning in a kind of normal fluctuation over a period of time. A chance event or something else that one cannot predict may trigger a giant fluctuation (a disorganizing process) that propels the system into a higher level of organization (Prigogine, Allen, & Herman, 1977). One cannot say the "normal" part, the organized part, is OK and the disorganized part is not. They are both part of the same process. If we are each in a process of expanding consciousness, and I submit that we are, then we are part of that process and must be present with it, attend to it, and live it, even if it appears in the form of disharmony, catastrophe, or disease.

In a recent review of the nursing research literature on health, I found that most of the research was based on the wellness-illness paradigm (Newman, in press). There were a few studies, however, that supported the transformational aspect of evolving consciousness. One in particular (Cowles, 1988) focused on the survivors of murder victims and the personal expansion of their world following this event: physical world expansion in terms of new environments and people; cognitive personal world expansion in terms of searching for the meaning of this event; emotional personal world expansion in terms of emotional response to the loss and the often disorganized physical world; and expansion into the victim's world, as the survivor assumed responsibility for protecting the victim's rights. This study is a powerful illustration of the personal expansion of consciousness that may take place as a result of a disorganizing event.

Many people have asked for an explanation of the relatedness of health as expanding consciousness to various catastrophic situations, for example, a child born with congenital anomalies, persons with Alzheimer's disease, or AIDS. The answer lies in extending the unit of analysis beyond the individual. In the above study, the focus was on the survivors of the murder victims. In terms of the child, one looks at the family of the child and what this experience means in terms of their consciousness. In regard to persons with AIDS, nurses who are working with persons with AIDS often report the tremendous expansion of the clients' consciousness in terms of their personal relationships and the meaning of their lives. We are tremendously saddened by the suffering that people go through, and none of us wants to go through that kind of suffering, but I submit it is better to go through the suffering and find oneself and the meaning of one's life and the meaning of one's relationships than not to have the experience and to go along on some superficial level.

What does this theory mean for nursing? If health is the expansion of consciousness and if disease is a manifestation of health as expanding consciousness, some would think that there is nothing for nursing to do. We can just sit back and allow it to happen. Not so. People need a partner in this process, particularly when they are suffering and do not find any meaning in what is going on. The thing that brings people to the attention of a nurse is that they are faced with situations that they do not know how to handle. They are at a turning point. Each of us at some time in our lives is brought to a point when the "old rules" do not work anymore, when what we have considered progress does not work anymore. We have done everything "right" about our health, but it still does not work—or we have done everything "right" about our relationships, but they still do not work. We come to a point when the old rules do not work and the task of life, *the crux of life,* is to learn

Shifting to Higher Consciousness

the new rules (Bateson, 1979; Young, 1976). This means learning how to transcend a situation that seems impossible, to find a new way to relate to things, and to discover the freedom that comes with transcending the old limitations.

That is where nursing comes in. Nursing can connect with the person when he or she is searching for new rules. By interacting with the person and sharing their consciousness, nurses can help to identify the pattern that is manifest. The light will go on—the insight into the pattern—and the person will see new possibilities. There is something right about the timing of the nurse-client meeting. It does not necessarily take a long time; it may take only a second. There is something about the timing of the nurse coming together with the client at that particularly critical point—sharing consciousness, moving apart, maybe coming back together in a kind of rhythmic fashion until the person can see his or her way clearly to greater freedom.

Part of what the nurse has to do is let go of wanting to control the situation. We have been taught to lead in the establishment of particular goals with the client and to work toward meeting those goals, and we are frustrated if the client wants to move in another direction. What we must do is let go of our own predetermined agenda and move in the direction of the client. We have to be able to allow the clients to make decisions that may go against the predominant values of the medical system. They may want to refuse treatment, they may want to go home to die, they may even decide to relinquish their responsibilities in the care of a child or an elderly parent. These are ways that may conflict with our own personal values, but we have to learn to let go of our own agenda and get in touch with where they are in this process of expanding consciousness and allow them to make their own choices and follow their own directions. One thing about the Prigogine theory that supports this difficult task is that the process is *not* predictable. When the system fluctuates in a giant way and assumes a new direction, it is not predictable. There are many different possibilities in terms of the direction the system may take, but one cannot predict ahead of time which one it will be. The task of the nurse is to be there for the patient as the possibilities present themselves and the client makes choices.

I began by talking about the way our world is changing: how the walls and barriers are breaking down, and cooperation among people is increasing. That is happening in the health care system as well, and nursing is in a position to be a predominant force in the giant fluctuation taking place. As we realize that a system based on manipulation and control does not work anymore, nursing will play an increasingly important part in the healing of our society. We are finding ways to become partners, partners with each other in a nonhierarchical network, partners with other professionals in the health field, and most of all, partners with clients. I am so glad that I'm a nurse in these times. Aren't you?

REFERENCES

Bahnson, C. B., & Bahnson, M. B. (1966). Role of the ego defenses: Denial and repression in the etiology of malignant neoplasm. *Annals of the New York Academy of Science, 125*(3), 827–845.

Bateson, G. (1979). *Mind and nature: A necessary unit.* New York: E. P. Dutton.

Bentov, I. (1978). *Stalking the wild pendulum.* New York: E. P. Dutton.

Bohm, D. (1980). *Wholeness and the implicate order.* London: Routledge & Kegan Paul.

Cowles, K. V. (1988). Personal world expansion for survivors of murder victims. *Western Journal of Nursing Research, 10*(6), 687–698.

Karagulla, S., & Kunz, D. (1989). *The chakras and the human energy fields.* Wheaton, IL: Theosophical Publishing.

Moss, R. (1981). *The I that is we.* Millbrae, CA: Celestial Arts.

Newman, M. A. (1975). The professional doctorate in nursing: A position paper. *Nursing Outlook, 23,* 704–706.

Newman, M. A. (1986). *Health as expanding consciousness.* St. Louis: C. V. Mosby.

Newman, M. A. (1990a). Professionalism: Myth or reality. In N. L. Chaska (Ed.). *The nursing profession: Turning points* (pp. 49–52). St. Louis: C. V. Mosby.

Newman, M. A. (1990b). Newman's theory of health as praxis. *Nursing Science Quarterly, 3*(1), 37–41.

Newman, M. A. (In press). Health conceptualizations and related research. *Annual Review of Nursing Research.*

Prigogine, I., Allen, P. M., & Herman, R. (1977). Long term trends and the evolution of complexity. In E. Laszlo & J. Bierman (Eds.). *Goals in a global community: The original background papers for goals for mankind,* Vol. 1 (pp. 1–63). New York: Pergamon.

Rogers, M. E. (1970). *An introduction to the theoretical basis of nursing.* Philadelphia: F. A. Davis.

Watson, J. (1989, June). *Future directions for substantive knowledge.* Paper presented at the National Forum on Doctoral Education in Nursing, Indianapolis, IN.

Wilber, K. (1979). Spectrum psychology, Part IV: Into the transpersonal. *Re-Vision, 2*(1), 65–72.

Young, A. E. (1976). *The reflexive universe: Evolution of consciousness.* San Francisco: Robert Briggs.

13

Application of Newman's Theory of Health: Pattern Recognition as Nursing Practice

Winnifred Gustafson

While we are immersed in the concerns of diagnosis-related groups, the nursing shortage, basic entry level, and differentiated practice issues, an even more significant development is going on in nursing today: the study of pattern and pattern recognition. Although pattern and pattern recognition have not yet become household words in our nursing vocabulary, they are by no means new. A group of nursing theorists has been wrestling with the concept of pattern for the past 15 years. The concept of pattern emerged out of the discoveries of quantum physics during the 1920s, and an extensive legacy of related thought has come down to us through Eastern philosophical teachings.

HISTORICAL OVERVIEW

Accustomed as we are to practicing nursing within the context of the scientific era, we may be surprised (and delighted) to find that scientists and scholars are increasingly conceding that traditional scientific methodologies are not the only path leading to knowledge about our world. Nor are they saying that it is enough just to add a warm element of caring on to scientific technology in order to make it more palatable for meaningful human experience. In fact, in the past 25 years, a school of thought known as the philosophy of science has emerged, which focuses on the shortcomings of the scientific method as we have known it (Keat & Urry, 1975).

Marilyn Ferguson, among others, has asserted that we have entered the postscientific era in which the ideas of cause and effect do not hold the same importance that they once did, but are merely one way of looking at things in order to find answers to particular questions asked at particular times (Ferguson, 1980). Our ideas about a "clockwork" mechanistic universe are broadening into an understanding of a universe that is relativistic and uncertain and that, indeed, contains everything past and present, known and unknown, here and there all at once!

We are well into this new way of thinking (many call it a new paradigm) in which informed, thoughtful scholars are writing about some very strange ideas. They are telling us that our understanding of space, time, and matter must be adjusted to the idea coming from modern physics that, at the subatomic level of investigation, things get less and less definite. As Capra (1975) explained, nature does not reveal isolated "basic building blocks," but rather appears as a complicated web of relations between the various parts of the whole. Mass is no longer associated with material substance, and particles are not seen as consisting of any basic "stuff," but as bundles of energy. In fact, what is going on at the subatomic level is influenced by the very presence of the observer.

When the macrocosmic levels are studied, similarly unsettling things are revealed. According to Einstein, there is no such thing as space (width, height, and depth) *and* time: there is only *space-time,* and it is a continuum. Zukov (1979) described it in this way:

> The special theory of relativity says that it is preferable, and more useful, to think in terms of a *static,* non-moving picture of space and time. This is the space-time continuum. In this static picture, the space-time continuum, events do not

develop, they just are. If we could view our reality in a four-dimensional way, we would see that everything that now seems to unfold before us with the passing of time, already exists *in toto,* painted as it were on the fabric of space-time. We would see all, the past, the present, and the future with one glance. Of course, this is only a mathematical proposition (isn't it?).

While this may sound pretty strange to our commonsense minds, some discoveries fit very well into a new way of thinking about our world, for instance, the hologram. In forming a hologram, light-waves are reflected off an object and recorded on a photographic film. When a laser beam of pure light is focused on the film, a seeming miracle takes place: the image of the object appears in three-dimensional form. The same image can be produced, although less clearly, from just a portion of the film. Karl Pribram, a neuroscientist at Stanford, proposed in 1969 that the hologram is a powerful model of our brain processes. David Bohm, a physicist at the University of London, proposed further that the organization of the universe may be holographic. Ferguson summarized their findings in this way:

> Our brains mathematically construct "concrete" reality by interpreting frequencies from another dimension, a realm of meaningful, patterned primary reality that transcends time and space. The brain is a hologram, interpreting a holographic universe (1980).

Although such ideas regarding the unity of mind and matter conflict with our accustomed way of discerning the world, an extensive legacy of such thought is found in the writings of Eastern philosophies and religions. While our Western world has been occupied with mind-body dualism, cause and effect, and scientific and technological advances, the Eastern perspective has portrayed the world in terms of cycles—of days, weeks, months, seasons, years, and ages of the gods—and the interconnectedness of people and all nature (Capra, 1975).

Now, what are we as pragmatic, action-oriented nurses to make of such ideas? Enter Margaret Newman! Newman has distilled the rarefied perspectives of a number of writers in the fields of philosophy of science, physics, neuroscience, and biochemistry and built upon the nursing theory of Martha Rogers to develop a theory of health that can illuminate our nursing practice.

NEWMAN'S THEORY OF HEALTH AS EXPANDING CONSCIOUSNESS

In presenting her theory, Newman (1986) contends that nursing interventions aimed at producing particular results become problematic when health is conceptualized as the expansion of consciousness in a universe of undivided wholeness. Instead of practicing in a traditional instrumental paradigm in which the nurse identifies what is wrong, why it is wrong, and what needs to be done to fix it, Newman offers a new paradigm. In this paradigm, the nurse enters into a partnership with the client to fulfill the mutual goal of participating in an authentic relationship, trusting that in the process both nurse and client will become healthier in the sense of attaining higher levels of consciousness. In the old paradigm, nursing process is divided into the separate steps of assessment, diagnosis, intervention, and evaluation. In the new paradigm, the process is one of pattern recognition in which there is a continuous merging of movement and understanding.

Newman's theory of health as expanding consciousness has been described as "not for the fainthearted" (Cowling, Pearson, & Silva, 1988). If so, then it follows that we are among the courageous today as we look at applying Newman's views on health and nursing in our practice. To me, however, her theory doesn't so much require special courage, but rather provides a useful and usable framework within which nursing can be practiced with confidence and creativity.

APPLICATION OF NEWMAN'S THEORY IN NURSING PRACTICE

Before I discuss the application of Newman's theory of health in my present practice as a parish nurse, let me briefly recap my own journey in nursing as a means of illustrating the connections I have made between theory and practice.

Like many others of my generation, I entered a diploma nursing program with an open mind as to what health, illness, and nursing were all about. Needless to say, my nursing education (in the early 50s) was all about illness. Health was something one took for granted, a sort of invisible baseline that was assumed to be there if one was active and productive. Illnesses, on the other hand, were named, described, and illustrated explicitly. There were lists of symptoms, medical treatments, nursing care procedures, and prognoses to be learned in detail. I remember the sudden realization early on in my nursing education that it was truly amazing that anyone was healthy at all in view of the multitudinous disease processes that abounded within the nursing texts and lectures—and, of course, on the hospital wards. I picked up the implicit message early that illness was "out there" just waiting for the time to attack. Illness was inevitable; health was just a temporary state.

As far as what we as nurses could do, we were led to believe that our task was to take care of patients, carry out doctor's orders, observe, and report (and run, not walk!). Keeping patients clean and comfortable; getting medications, treatments, and charting done on time; transcribing and carrying out physicians' orders; keeping ward order and hospital routine—all of these were simply the givens of nursing. Nursing interventions and patient outcomes were not even mentioned. Nursing prowess was seen in unswerving action, perseverance, and endurance in completing heavy assignments—replete with interruptions and distractions—before the next shift came on.

I do, however, remember bright spots of affirmation for "good observation." (I can still hear our stern but kindly Miss Jones saying, "Very good, you were very observant.") The need for seeing, hearing, smelling, touching, feeling, and *knowing* was continually reinforced so that even as the hospital-medical expectations of completing tasks on time were fulfilled, the nursing expectation of being observant on behalf of the patients' well-being was also fulfilled—although often at an intuitive, even subconscious level.

All old nurses have stories to tell about this mysterious intuitive knowing that emerged at times in seemingly inexplicable ways. My first formal awareness of the ability of nurse and patient to intuit a situation, came during my first year as a new graduate. During the small hours of the night, while talking briefly with a wakeful patient, I learned that he had a vague, uneasy feeling that something was wrong, that he might even die. Since he was in the hospital for ulcer treatment (before the days of cimetidine), I checked him and his vital signs often as the morning ward activity picked up. Finally, in a burst of concern and courage, I called his physician at 5 A.M. to report the patient's sense of "impending doom" (as the texts called it then), even though I could not detect any measurable symptoms. The physician came in early, but his exam and tests did not reveal any serious problem either. The next night, as I came on duty, I heard about the shock crisis that had suddenly developed that day, at which time the man was rushed to surgery to locate and stop the source of internal hemorrhage. Here clearly was a case where the physical symptoms (or lack of them) gave incomplete—even misleading information—about the man's unfolding situation, which he and I had sensed intuitively during the early morning hours.

Since then, experiences revealing the powerful sense of exchange and interaction that can occur between patients and nurses even during the briefest encounters have accumulated. It wasn't until much later, when I was writing my master's thesis on caring (Gustafson, 1981), that it occurred to me that the injection, pill, dressing change, or whatever it was that brought me into a hospital room—as important as it might be—was often only a sort of permit to enter the special world of concern that a person was experiencing just then. I was awakened to the fact, too, that such interactions opened up windows of understanding about life for both of us, nurse and patient.

As you can see, I am a latecomer to nursing theory. (In fact, as a returning RN student, I was just learning that nursing theory existed at about the time that Newman was publishing *Theory Development in Nursing* (1979). Since then, I have learned that nursing theory truly serves as a powerful description and explanation of what we are doing when we are nursing effectively. When it comes to theory development and theory-based practice, we are all in this together—thinkers and doers alike.

While I have learned a great deal and gained important insights from the works of all our nursing theorists, Margaret Newman's theory of health is the most helpful to me in making sense of my past nursing experience, as well as the most useful in my present practice as a parish nurse. I have found that for practical purposes (and isn't that what it all comes down to?), nursing theory is most applicable to nursing practice when it enlightens our highest levels of conceptualization. Newman's theory does just that by dealing with the all-embracing ideas of space, time, movement, and consciousness. With such a comprehensive perspective of our universe, we can perceive anew how we fit in this universe as people who share in all the various exigencies of daily living. By first internalizing the concepts and terminology at the highest, most inclusive level—by making the paradigm shift—our perceptions are transformed regarding health, illness, and nursing.

Making the Paradigm Shift

While struggling with how to make the idea of the paradigm shift more accessible to our pragmatic nursing world, I was recently surprised by a colorful illustration projected on the wall of my home-office (a.k.a. kitchen-dining area). I had taken time out the day before to wash and rearrange the colored glass collection on the window sash, among them a clear glass prism, somewhat chipped and scratched, but intact overall. Now glancing up from the typewriter, I was delighted by colorful bands of light decorating the cupboard doors in a surprising new display of illumination. In replacing the prism, I had changed its position and angle so that the sun's rays were refracted through it in a new manifestation of color intensity and design.

I see this as an illustration that even as nurses feeling somewhat used and scarred by our experiences within prevailing medical settings, we can align ourselves anew to catch the rays of enlightenment that will illuminate our understanding of life, health, and nursing. While we may often appear to be *doing* many of the traditional nursing activities in the everyday world of nursing, the *outcomes* will be surprisingly creative and energizing as we authentically interact with others within a new frame of reference.

Another way of grasping the idea of the paradigm shift comes from Palmer's (1983) description of "wholesight." We have been taught to maintain "one-eyed" lives and rely largely on the eye of the mind to form our image of reality. In an effort to counteract the flawed nature of a "mind-made" world, we often work at opening the eye of the heart to see a world that includes love and caring. But as Palmer asks: "How shall we bring together these two lines of sight? How shall we use both the eyes of the mind and the heart to create not a blurry double image but one world, in all its dimensions, healed and made whole?"

As nurses, we have traditionally sought to use both the eyes of the mind and the heart, opting to live with the resultant blurred double image in an effort to survive in a medical-technological environment while endeavoring to maintain a caring stance. Newman's theory serves as a means for attaining wholesight, a perspective of the world in which mind and heart can unite.

As we work to shift to the new paradigm and maintain wholesight in our nursing practice, we will need to share our experiences along the way. A good starting point is understanding how we view ourselves and our clients. In my parish nursing, I have sought to transform my view of the nurse-client relationship on the basis of Newman's (1986) illustration of the holographic model of intervention. As she explains, when two people interact, waves of energy radiate from each person and intersect with the other's pattern, thus becoming an interference pattern that in turn becomes part of the pattern of each. Instead of conceptualizing people in the usual way as single and separate vertical or horizontal entities, I re-envision ourselves as concentric circles of energy. Rather than thinking of interpersonal relationships as attempts to reach from me (here) to you (there), I accept that we are already connected by virtue of our sharing space within a given environment, community, interest area, and/or shared thought process.

It sometimes seems that our patterns merely brush by each other, as in a grocery check-out line or in an elevator ride. Oftentimes there is greater intersection of pattern, ranging in degree from small-talk encounters to the deeply blended intersections of pattern within our significant relationships. In the context of nursing practice, the potential for this deeper intersection of pattern exists even within the briefest encounters. If, as Newman asserted, the task of nursing intervention is pattern recognition, then we must reach for a clearer understanding of this process, and the practicalities of who can do it, and when and where it can occur.

Who Can "Do" Pattern Recognition?

In addressing the *who* of pattern recognition, Carper's (1978) study on patterns of knowing in nursing indicated that pattern recognition is indeed a "natural" for nurses. Carper found that nurses use four types of interrelated and interdependent knowing in their practice of nursing: empirical (factual, descriptive, and ultimately explanatory), esthetic, personal, and ethical. As she summarized, "Nursing thus depends on the scientific knowledge of human behavior in health and in illness, the esthetic perception of significant human experiences, a personal understanding of the unique individuality of the self, and the capacity to make choices within concrete situations involving particular moral judgments." Of these patterns of knowing, Carper saw the component of personal knowledge as most essential to understanding the meaning of health in terms of an individual's well-being: "Personal knowledge is concerned with the knowing, encountering, and actualizing of the concrete individual self. One does not know *about* the self; one strives simply to *know* the self."

Allport (1961) supported the perceptual capacity for pattern recognition that is inherent in humans and discussed the qualifications for being a good judge of personality. He concluded that the patterned perception of personality is the comprehension of organization, with the aid of inference, under a sustained interest in the structure of the other personality.

From another perspective, Gardner (1983) looked at the natural qualities that enable us to detect patterns in our associations with others. Along with intelligences in the areas of linguistics, music, logic-mathematics, spatial relationships, and body movement, Gardner included the personal intelligences of the intrapersonal and interpersonal. He cited evidence that one set of cortical regions, located in the dorsal or parietal region of the cortex, seems critical for surveillance, attention, and arousal. Its injury results in indifference and in the loss of a sense of caring about oneself. A contrasting set of cortical regions, located in the ventral or temporal region of the cortex, seems critical for the identification of stimuli, for new learning, and for appropriate emotional responding. Lesions in this latter area produce a lack of concern with external stimuli and, accordingly, inappropriate responses toward other individuals.

Gardner drew parallels between these forms of brain impairment and the two types of personal intelligences (intrapersonal and interpersonal). He pointed out that although personal intelligences may be rooted in biology, they are expressed differently across cultures. He inferred that knowledge of self and others may be at a higher level or more integrated form of intelligence, "one more at the behest of the culture and of historical factors, one more truly emergent, one that ultimately comes to control and to regulate more 'primary orders' of intelligence."

Since knowing ourselves and others through pattern perception is an innate and essential human cognitive ability, Newman's call for pattern methodology is indeed timely as we move into a new paradigm of health and nursing. As in all aptitudes and abilities, however, it may be that some people have an advantage in developing expertise in pattern recognition.

According to the Myers-Briggs Type Indicator (1987), individuals have a preference for acquiring information through either the sensing or intuitive functions. In the sensing function, seeing, hearing, and the other senses tell us what is present and happening inside and outside of ourselves. Sensing types tend to accept and work with what is given in the present moment, and thus are realistic and practical. On the other hand, intuitive people seek the meanings, relationships, and possibilities that go beyond the information gained through the senses. Intuitive types look at the big picture and try to grasp the essential patterns.

While nursing traditionally emphasized and rewarded the sensing function in nursing practice, contemporary nursing increasingly calls for the intuitive function in drawing nursing diagnoses from assessment data. Benner's (1984) work on analyzing exemplars of expert nursing practice emphasized the necessity of drawing upon both the sensing and intuiting functions. Benner (1989) further concluded, "Pattern recognition is an essential component of nursing expertise. We need to make it a more legitimate and visible element of our practice."

Nursing is not alone in this recent effort to focus on pattern-recognition abilities. Taylor (1990) contended that in the search for creating artificial intelligence, one of the greatest problems is figuring out how humans recognize patterns and how they can relate prior knowledge to novel situations: "Unlike most computers, which send data and instructions single file between a single memory, each processor shares in storing a tiny bit of many units of information. The system of connections between these processors—the "neural network"—may be the secret of humans' distinctive cognitive abilities."

When and Where Can Pattern Recognition Occur?

If the task in nursing intervention is pattern recognition (Newman, 1986), it follows that we can see indicators of this modality wherever and whenever nurses and clients come together. If pattern recognition is an essential component of expert nursing (Benner, 1989), we can find evidence for pattern recognition at the very heart of our nursing experiences.

Three perspectives on pattern recognition are found in the nursing literature. First, Benner (1984, 1989) raised nursing consciousness regarding the ways that experienced nurses synthesize their knowledge about health, disease symptoms, medical treatment modalities, and nursing interventions in order to understand a client's unique "whole" situation. She documented many exemplars where nurses acted on behalf of clients, alerted through a "sixth sense" that emerged beyond their own usual and expected levels of perception and knowledge.

Another aspect of pattern recognition has been delineated by Newman (1987), Moch (1988), and Jonsdottir (1988) where information from clients was examined for pattern configurations and reflected back to the client for verification and discussion. In this praxis-oriented research, interviewees gained insight into their own patterns and action possibilities (Newman, 1990).

A third approach to pattern recognition grows out of Newman's (1966) study on identifying and meeting patient needs in short-span nurse-patient relationships where effective communication was found to be the basis for quality nursing decisions and actions. Since then, Newman's work attests that something more significant occurs between client and nurse which goes beyond good communication techniques:

> The essence of nursing is not doing or manipulating but is being open to whatever arises in the interaction with the client. It is being fully present with an unconditional acceptance of the client's experience. The nurse offers her/his whole self so that the client can resonate with an authentic person. The nurse is like a tuning fork through which the client can begin to resonate with the consciousness of the universe (1989).

It is this latter intriguing and mystifying perspective on pattern recognition that has served as the focal point for exploration within my present nursing practice experiences.

"Doing" Pattern Recognition

This exploratory look at pattern recognition as nursing intervention has taken place in a parish nurse practice setting. Gloria Dei Lutheran Church, Duluth, Minnesota, is one of about 150 churches nationwide that have followed the example and leadership of retired Lutheran minister Granger Westberg, who started the parish nurse program seven years ago at Lutheran General Hospital in Park Ridge, Illinois (Westberg, 1987). Gloria Dei's pastor and congregation share the holistic view that the soul and body are inseparable components in health. They base their parish nurse program on the belief that churches should renew their historical tasks of teaching, preaching, and healing.

The program, nearly three years old, serves people free of charge both within the congregation and the community in which the church is located. The parish nurse is available to people of all ages; however, about three-fourths of the clientele are in their 80s and 90s. As parish nurse, I am contacted most often to help people make the transition between various levels of independence and dependence and link them to available community services.

The newly developing parish nurse practice served well for this inquiry into pattern recognition because appointments were usually arranged ahead of time, there was often driving time that could be used to refocus thinking in preparation for a visit, and the schedule was arranged so that there were minimal time constraints for an initial visit. The initial visit in particular was open-ended and free-flowing according to the needs and wishes of the client.

In preparation for visits with people requesting a parish nurse visit, I sought to internalize Newman's description of pattern recognition:

> This occurs . . . by going into ourselves and getting in touch with our own pattern and through it in touch with the pattern of the person or persons with whom we are interacting . . . (The) process of focusing is a helpful starting point. This process involves directed concentration on oneself, more specifically on the feelings one is aware of in the body. It may be a heaviness in the heart or stomach area, a pain in the shoulders or lower back, or something far more diffuse. The task is to concentrate on that feeling, to get in touch with it, and try to explicate it by naming it. If the first name you give it does not "feel" right, you stay with it and continue to name it until your identification of the feeling coincides with the deeper nonverbal message of your body. When this congruence is reached, there is usually a total relaxing shift that occurs in your body similar to that experienced when you finally remember something that you have been blocking on. This process of focusing and relaxing releases energy for growth even when you are not conscious of what growth is occurring, and this is true when you practice the process with someone else. If you are the facilitator, you are acting like the reference beam in the hologram, making it possible for the interference pattern to emerge and for pattern recognition to occur (Newman, 1986).

After each initial visit during the first year of my parish nurse practice, I recorded client assessments using the dimensions of person-environment interaction developed by the nurse theorist group of the North American Nursing Diagnosis Association. These dimensions (Newman, 1986) are defined as follows: (1) exchanging: interchanging matter and energy between person and environment, and transforming energy from one form to another; (2) communicating: interchanging information from one system to another; (3) relating: connecting with other persons and the environment; (4) valuing: assigning worth; (5) choosing: selecting of one or more alternatives; (6) moving: rhythmic alternating between activity and rest; (7) perceiving: receiving and interpreting information; (8) feeling: sensing physical and intuitive awareness; and (9) knowing: personal recognizing of self and world.

Data were organized as clusters of client information from which deductions were drawn regarding the client's pattern. For example, following an unstructured initial visit in which the client conversationally chatted about her concerns, I recorded Mrs. L.'s assessment data in this way:

Exchanging

- Respiration, circulation, nutrition, elimination are as Mrs. L. says, "all very good for age 93."
- Avoids fatty, spicy foods because they don't agree.
- Always eats a good breakfast, a light lunch, and fixes meat and vegetables for supper.
- Some incontinence when she waits too long to start up the stairs to the bathroom.
- Takes Lasix 40 mg. five days a week; has negotiated with physician that she can skip days when she is going out.

Communicating

- Discusses ideas as well as relating events.
- Enjoys reading newspaper and large-print books.
- Conversational in person and on phone; voice sounds somewhat strained but projects clearly; hard of hearing but not sure she is ready for a hearing aid yet.

Relating

- Speaks fondly of family relationships and get-togethers.
- Feels sad and lonely when she thinks of family and friends who have died.
- Appreciates being honored as a senior member of the congregation.
- Misses her former experiences of knowing everyone in the church, although she is glad for the young people who are joining the church lately.
- Wishes for more one-to-one visits in her home where she can be an active participant in the conversation.

Valuing

- Values faith in God, Swedish Lutheran traditions, cooperation among people, sensitivity to the feelings of others, orderliness, hospitality, mementos and memories of the past.

Choosing

- Decided to request parish nurse visit to discuss hearing loss, occasional stress incontinence, and potential need for homemaking and personal care assistance.
- Chooses to live in home built by her father regardless of inconvenience of stairs ("but I get my exercise that way"), being alone much of time, and concern of others for her safety.

Moving

- Walks slowly and carefully with cane.
- Rests in rocking chair when not otherwise occupied.
- Naps several times a day "while watching TV;" sleeps all night usually.
- Demonstrates careful use of stairs, holding handrail; has cane for upstairs use, also one for basement use.
- Goes to church and Sunday dinners with friends and family who provide rides and assist with walking.

- Takes taxi for some appointments ("the drivers can be very helpful").
- Fell on her way into the beauty salon last month ("just some bruises"), even more careful now; "I learned my lesson not to try to do it on my own."

Perceiving

- Perceives the world changing from the solid and stable past ("but we have to go along with it, what else can we do?").
- Reflects changes in self-esteem related to difficulties in group conversations.
- Perceives opinions of others differing from her own because of her career background (widowed in late 30s, no children) as a legal secretary.
- Perceives vision as "adequate" with bifocals and magnifiers.

Feeling

- Aware that others have experienced God's love and care through her past hospital visitation activities.
- Aware of the needs of shut-ins from her own experience now, but feels regrets that she didn't do more for others when she was younger ("I didn't understand what they were going through").
- Feels joint stiffness and pain especially in the morning ("but it eases up as the day goes along so I won't complain").
- Is aware and thankful for her general state of good health.

Knowing

- Knows what to do and who to call for assistance.
- Knows that others are sincere in desire to help her, but knows her own reluctance to accept help. "I like when people offer, then I can accept or refuse as the case may be."
- Recollects the past in detail, but also knows the news of today.
- Says, "I know that God knows when my time will be up, I just need to be ready for what He has planned."

Emerging pattern

- Enjoys a sense of continuity and wholeness about her life.
- Appreciates her individuality as it compares and contrasts with others.
- Integrates health changes of aging into her personal hygiene, home safety modifications, and social contact style.

Although this pattern summary appeared very broad as initially stated, it has proven surprisingly enlightening to me in the past two and a half years. Mrs. L. and I have continued to visit, sometimes briefly at church or on the phone, and sometimes at greater length in her home or when driving together for doctor appointments. A consistency of pattern is evident in the way that Mrs. L. experiences health changes (cataract surgery and intraocular implant, hearing aid adjustment, and several arthritis flare-ups) and changes in her living arrangements (home health aide assistance, delivered noon meals, and more frequent overnight visits from concerned out-of-town nieces). The initial pattern statement has provided insight for me as her facilitator, and she in turn expresses understanding and appreciation for the unique person she is. With privileged perception of her pattern, I sense that I am walking with her, learning about life from her.

Through assessment of the dimensions of person-environment interaction, and a statement of the emerging pattern that I perceive, I have a valuable point of reference about the client. This knowledge, although not necessarily predictive, affords me a sense of tranquillity as I share in the ongoing health concerns of my clients. The usefulness of pattern recognition becomes clearer as I review and compare the patterns of several people. For example, my notes on Mrs. D. indicate that she is "absorbed with home and memories of the past" and "interacts with others and environment to the extent necessary for maintaining integrity of self and home." Two years after writing this, I appreciate the appropriateness of Mrs. D.'s actions in renting out rooms to two students so that, although she much prefers privacy and quiet, she can remain in her home a while longer.

My notes regarding Mr. P. indicate that he is "enmeshed within home and secluded life-style through memories and commitments of the past, open to friendly overtures of selected people who respect his family history, and moving slowly and hesitantly toward a change in living arrangements (but waiting for a decision to be made for him through external circumstances such as injury or surgery)." Six months after writing this pattern statement, I called Mr. P. one day at a prearranged time, found that he had slid to the floor from his chair and was not able to get up, thereby setting in motion the forces for his move into a nursing home. After an initial period of physical therapy and non-steroidal anti-inflammatory drug treatment, Mr. P. was slowly but surely arranging to sell his home to a buyer skilled in upgrading and renovating houses.

Another client, Mrs. A., has a lifetime history of emotional concerns and social service support. My notes on her indicate she has an "erratic rest and activity pattern and is consuming assistance, resources, information, food, and medication in extraordinary amounts in order to maintain a sense of equilibrium that steadies her diffusive and wide-ranging thought patterns and communication style." I am learning a great deal about pattern recognition from Mrs. A. as I seek to offer her unconditional acceptance during our visits. She in turn is expansive in her appreciation that I will listen to her "let off steam" periodically. By focusing on my own pattern during our "talks," Mrs. A.'s diffusive pattern gradually seems to become more focused, often enabling and empowering her to act productively.

While an assessment framework proved very helpful in my early efforts to recognize patterns, I soon found that an increasingly busy schedule kept me from writing up detailed reports following each initial client visit. But as Newman (1986) observed, pattern recognition is more a matter of being able to read one's own pattern than of collecting information external to oneself. As we become sensitive to our thoughts, feelings, and visualizations, and learn to trust them, we become adept at doing so quickly—even instantly—as we interact with others (1989).

As we seek to understand and share the process of pattern recognition, there can be an amount of hesitancy and embarrassment in revealing what works for us—or what has worked for us in the past—for fear that it sounds too subjective or trivial. In reflecting upon my past hospital nursing experiences, I am aware that I enjoyed my work most and felt most effective when I was able to clear my mind and approach patients with a sense of expectancy, readiness, and availability for whatever would occur. Going back to my days as a student, I believe that pinning my cap in place (in the days of required nursing caps) originally served as a signal for this mind set.

Seeking a more explicit explanation of how I achieve the proper mind set for pattern recognition, I find that I use a brief thought-prayer to give up any blockage or haziness that I am consciously or unconsciously bringing into the situation and replace it with a sense of curiosity about how the situation will turn out. In learning about pattern recognition, we must watch for points where we feel that pattern recognition occurs and how the desired mind set can be renewed when the ability seems to slip away. For regaining the proper perspective when my mind wanders or I begin to feel bored, I find it helpful to visualize a space-view of the earth and follow it down to our continent, area and city, and then down to the specific address where I am meeting with a client. In this mental process, I again grasp a sense of the emerging pattern that is unfolding in space, time, and movement as a part of the greater universe.

As far as watching for points where pattern recognition occurs, my experience is that clients are ready to connect anytime that we as nurses are ready. For example, recently I gathered up a dozen bright plants in my car and proceeded to make as many friendly calls as I could from mid-morning to supper-time. Since I usually call before dropping in on people, this was a new experience and I wondered how it would go. No problem. As I introduced myself to Mrs. J. whom I had not yet met in person, she interrupted me with, "Oh, you're the nurse—do you have a cure for arthritis today?" and away we went for an hour of delightful sharing. When I came to Mrs. K.'s door, she peered up at me through her thick glasses and said, "Is that you? I was just going to dial your number. Come in, we'll have lunch and talk." Later, finding Mrs. N.'s door ajar, I looked in as I knocked and called out to her. She readily responded, "Oh, yes, I need a nurse for sure today," and with no other warm-up, she launched out upon her sea of concerns.

So, is pattern recognition useful and feasible in nursing? By all means. As nurses we have often unconsciously engaged in it while doing our nursing tasks, not realizing that we were involved in something so significant to the ongoing unfolding of the universe!

REFERENCES

Allport, G. W. (1961). *Pattern and growth in personality.* New York: Holt, Rinehart, & Winston.

Benner, P. (1984). *From novice to expert.* Menlo Park, CA: Addison-Wesley Publishing Company.

Benner, P. (1989). Commentary. *American Journal of Nursing, 89,* 503.

Capra, F. (1975). *The tao of physics.* New York: Bantam Books.

Carper, B. (1978). Fundamental patterns of knowing in nursing. *Advances in Nursing Science, 1*(1), 13–23.

Cowling, W. R., Pearson, B. D., & Silva, M. C. (1988). Book reviews. *Nursing Science Quarterly, 1*(3), 133–138.

Ferguson, M. (1980). *The aquarian conspiracy.* Los Angeles: J. P. Tarcher.

Gardner, H. (1983). *Frames of mind, the theory of multiple intelligences.* New York: Basic Books.

Gustafson, W. (1981). *An analysis of the concept of caring toward the testable descriptive theory.* Unpublished master's thesis, University of Minnesota.

Jonsdottir, H. (1988). *Health patterns of clients with chronic obstructive pulmonary disease.* Unpublished master's thesis, University of Minnesota.

Keat, R., & Urry, J. (1975). *Social theory as science.* London: Routledge & Kegan Paul.

Moch, S. (1988). *Health in illness: Experiences with breast cancer* (Doctoral dissertation, University of Minnesota). *Dissertation Abstracts International, 50,* 47b.

Myers, I. B. (1987). *Introduction to type.* Palo Alta, CA: Consulting Psychologists Press.

Newman, M. A. (1966). Identifying patient needs in short-span nurse-patient relationships. *Nursing Forum, 5*(1), 76–86.

Newman, M. A. (1979). *Theory development in nursing.* Philadelphia: F. A. Davis.

Newman, M. A. (1986). *Health as expanding consciousness.* St. Louis: C. V. Mosby.

Newman, M. A. (1987). Patterning. In M. Duffy & N. J. Pender (Eds.). *Conceptual issues in health promotion: Report of proceedings of a wingspread conference* (pp. 36–50). Indianapolis: Sigma Theta Tau.

Newman, M. A. (1989). The spirit of nursing. *Holistic Nursing Practice, 3*(3), 1–6.

Newman, M. A. (1990). Newman's theory of health as praxis. *Nursing Science Quarterly, 3*(1), 37–41.

Palmer, P. J. (1983). *To know as we are known.* San Francisco: Harper & Row.

Taylor, R. (1990, March). So human a machine. *Update.* University of Minnesota.

Westberg, G. (1987). *The parish nurse.* Park Ridge, IL: Parish Nurse Resource.

Zukov, G. (1979). *The dancing Wu Li masters.* New York: Bantam Books.

14

The Gift: Applying Newman's Theory of Health in Nursing Practice

Kathleen A. Kalb

> "Every experience of life is a gift,
> to be claimed and learned from."
> Margaret Newman, 1986

The application of Newman's theory of health as expanding consciousness is truly a gift to nursing practice, for it empowers the nurse to engage in the process of pattern recognition with clients. In this process, the nurse and the client become partners in a relationship characterized by negotiation, reciprocity, and empowerment. This mutually rewarding relationship is the essence of Newman's theory of health as praxis and will be the focus of this chapter on the application of Newman's theory in the clinical management of preterm labor.

NURSING PRACTICE AS PATTERN RECOGNITION

The professional practice of nursing under Newman's theory of health as expanding consciousness necessitates commitment to authentic relationships with the clients. According to this emerging paradigm (Newman, 1986), the nurse engages in pattern recognition with clients, interacting with and assisting clients to determine the total meaning of their experiences. In this paradigm of health, the nurse-client relationship is based on pattern recognition and is defined by the individual wholeness of the client in interaction with his or her environment. Nursing practice is directed toward the recognition of this person-environment pattern of interaction and is operationalized in the nurse's authentic involvement with the client in a mutual and reciprocal relationship. It is in the enhanced understanding of the client's underlying pattern that the nurse and the client become partners and participants in experiencing the pattern of consciousness formed by their interaction.

In this new paradigm of health, the client is viewed as an autonomous participant and the health professional is viewed as a therapeutic partner (Ferguson, 1980). The client is respected and experienced as an integrated whole, the interaction of mind, body, and environment. In this interaction, the body is seen as a dynamic system, a field of energy within other fields. Health, in this paradigm, involves a search for patterns; information in this search primarily comes from the client's subjective reports and the professional's intuition. Wholeness, according to Ferguson (1980), originates in an attitude: an acceptance of life's uncertainties, a willingness to accept responsibility for habits, a way of perceiving and dealing with stress, participation in satisfying human relationships, a sense of purpose. A holistic view of the client in the new paradigm of health recognizes the relational, patterned, and unitary characteristics of the client as an integrated whole.

Initially, an assessment framework consistent with this paradigm of health may assist the nurse in the process of pattern recognition. Based on the following assumptions: (1) that the pattern of a person is unitary and maintains its identity through continuous change, and (2) that the human energy field and the environmental energy field are in constant interaction with each other, this assessment framework specifically addresses nine dimensions of person-environment interaction to be considered by the nurse—exchanging, communicating, relating, valuing, choosing, moving, perceiving, feeling, and knowing. These dimensions are manifestations of the unitary pattern, and they characterize the interaction of the person in his or her environment (Newman, 1984). These dimensions have been modified and described by Newman (1986) as: (1) exchanging: the interchanging matter and energy between persons and environment and transforming energy from one form to another; (2) communicating: interchanging information from one system to another; (3) relating: connecting with other persons and the environment; (4) valuing: assigning worth; (5) choosing: selecting of one or more alternatives; (6) moving: rhythmic alternating between activity and rest; (7) perceiving: receiving and interpreting information; (8) feeling: sensing physical and intuitive awareness; and (9) knowing: personal recognizing of self and world.

The meaning of the underlying pattern of the person-environment interaction may be assessed using the nine dimensions of this framework. The emergence of this pattern of person-environment interaction can then be viewed as movement-space-time patterns of consciousness (Newman, 1986). Therefore, information is assessed by the nurse with the client in a search for the underlying pattern of the individual in interaction with his or her environment. In this emerging paradigm of health, pattern recognition becomes the essence of nursing practice (Newman, 1986).

This paradigm of pattern was applied in a program of care developed with pregnant women hospitalized for complications of maternal-fetal health. High risk pregnancy is defined as the existence of adverse physiological manifestations of maternal-fetal health occurring between 12 and 38 weeks of gestation. For pregnant women, the experience of high risk pregnancy may represent the "chance element and/or critical event" that yields alterations in the physical and social world in the form of behavioral change. These alterations in the individual's pattern of health require energy from the environment to produce a higher level of organization and a new level of consciousness (Newman, 1986). Through the intervention of pattern recognition, the nurse caring for women experiencing high risk pregnancy may provide the source of the environmental energy that can lead to the expansion of consciousness.

As co-participants in the experience of high risk pregnancy, both the nurse and the client have the opportunity to determine the unique meaning of their interaction in their pattern of connectedness. The nurse facilitates the woman's ability to recognize her own pattern in the experience of high risk pregnancy. Pattern recognition enables the pregnant woman to integrate the meaning of her experience as part of her evolving pattern. The pattern of her unborn child is also a part of the woman's unitary pattern to be recognized and integrated. This "pattern within a pattern" is explicated in the experience of pregnancy.

In the traditional paradigm of health, the management of high risk pregnancy is focused on the treatment of the adverse physiological manifestation of maternal-fetal health. When this focus on treatment occurs in isolation from the totality of the woman's experience of pregnancy, the woman's pattern of the whole may be negated. By engaging in an authentic relationship with the woman experiencing high risk pregnancy, the nurse is able to integrate the meaning of this interaction as part of the nurse's own pattern of consciousness, a pattern that may then be shared in encounters with other women experiencing high risk pregnancies.

The nurse, engaged in the practice of pattern recognition and committed to this relational paradigm of health as expanding consciousness, experiences integration and growth through interaction with clients. What is sensed in terms of pattern becomes a function of the nurse's own level of awareness, sensitivity to self, and point of view (Newman, 1986). This process of transformation through the experience of pattern recognition is the essence of nursing practice in the new paradigm. This is nursing practice as praxis, the "gift" we give ourselves as we become partners in health through negotiation, reciprocity, and empowerment with our clients and colleagues.

PATTERN RECOGNITION IN PREGNANCY

The condition of high risk pregnancy in the new paradigm of health becomes a process to be experienced as part of the pattern of the whole; not as an entity to be alienated from the self or cured. Rather, in the experience of caring for the woman with a high risk pregnancy, the emphasis is on the whole and not the parts. In a holistic approach to preterm labor, for example, the nurse does not focus on only the contracting uterus, the part of the body manifesting a complication and alteration of pregnancy. Instead, the nurse considers the contracting uterus as a part of the whole client in holistic interaction with her body, mind, and environment. The uterine contractions are merely indications of a pattern of relationships that reveal the underlying process of the whole in that specific moment in time, space, and movement.

Newman's theory of health as pattern has special relevance for women experiencing high risk pregnancy. Women are generally diagnosed with a high risk pregnancy when fetal health is jeopardized. Frequently, the gestating mother alone is able to be the conduit through which care can be delivered to the unborn child. This places the pregnant woman in a situation where she must choose how she will care for her unborn child prenatally.

Pregnancy is an acute process. The period of gestation usually lasts approximately nine months (a term pregnancy is defined as lasting 38 to 42 weeks). However, the implications of pregnancy are chronic in the continuing experience of parenting. This situation of acute chronicity is unique in pregnancy as the limited period of gestation sets the stage for the evolving pattern of interaction between the pregnant woman and her unborn child. This sustained interaction of the unborn child's pattern within the pregnant woman's pattern characterizes the lifelong mother-child relationship.

Pregnancy also presents a unique opportunity for pattern recognition. The uniqueness in pregnancy of experiencing a pattern within a pattern is unparalleled. The pattern of the maternal-fetal unit is characterized by the pattern of the unborn child within the pattern of the pregnant woman within the pattern of the family and community. In a high risk pregnancy, pattern recognition becomes a complex and dynamic interaction of the unborn child's pattern of person-environment interaction within the pregnant woman's pattern. Truly, pattern recognition in high risk pregnancy is a significant challenge for nursing practice.

Women experience profound alterations in their patterns of person-environment interaction during pregnancy. These alterations are related to their experiences of pregnancy, as well as to the iatrogenically induced alterations associated with the diagnosis of high risk pregnancy. When hospitalization is required for the assessment and management of high risk pregnancy, these alterations are experienced in triplicate as the alterations of hospitalization are superimposed upon the alterations necessitated in the management of high risk pregnancy, as superimposed upon the experience of pregnancy. These alterations may be enumerated in the four manifestations of pattern described by Newman (1986) as aspects of the total pattern of an individual's person-environment interaction: movement, time, space, and consciousness.

MANIFESTATIONS OF PATTERN IN PREGNANCY

The iatrogenically induced alterations that occur when women are hospitalized for the treatment and management of high risk pregnancy are superimposed upon the alterations that pregnancy alone induces in a woman's lived experience of her pattern. Alterations created by pregnancy, for example, may include changes in a woman's pattern of movement, her kinesthetic consciousness. Since it is through movement that we expand our knowledge of ourselves, others, and the environment (Newman, 1986), the alterations related to movement during the experience of pregnancy are important considerations in the pregnant woman's expansion of consciousness.

Pregnant women move more slowly, especially as pregnancy progresses and their weight and size increase. The hormones of pregnancy alter a woman's perception and she feels tired and fatigued, especially in the first and third trimesters of pregnancy. These perceptions of fatigue may have significant effects upon the woman's ability to continue her previous pattern of interaction with the environment and the control she has previously been able to maintain in the quality of her interactions. The awareness of her unborn child's pattern of activity and movement throughout the day, as well as the circadian pattern of uterine activity and contractions, may alter a woman's perception of her own rhythmicity and movement. Because the pattern of movement reflects the overall organization of the thought and feeling processes of a person (Newman, 1986), the experience of pregnancy also alters a woman's perception of space-time.

The pregnant woman's perception of time is frequently altered as she anticipates the birth of her child. "This is taking forever," are words frequently expressed by pregnant women. This alteration is experienced particularly in the third trimester when movement also slows down and increased fatigue is common. As an indicator of the personal tempo or basic rhythm of a person, the perception of time in pregnancy is likely to be experienced as the way the woman has experienced her life, and "is inextricably linked to space and movement" (Newman, 1986).

As pregnancy continues and the unborn child develops, the woman's size and shape is altered and becomes larger. This increased body space frequently results in an altered self-image. It is also interesting to consider the language we use to describe pregnancy, in particular the notion of the "expected date of confinement," the due date. This notion of restricted movement and the perception of altered space during the experience of pregnancy are images explicitly created by our language.

Consciousness, according to Newman (1990), is a manifestation of the evolving pattern of person-environment interaction. Defined as the informational capacity of the system, consciousness is described as the ability of the person to interact with his or her environment. The awareness of new sensations within the pregnant woman's body, the feelings of fetal movement, the hormonal fluctuations, the alterations of her own bodily rhythms (for example, in the sleep-wake cycle), and the synchronicity (or lack of synchronicity) of self with the unborn child are all manifestations of an altered perception of consciousness experienced in pregnancy. Alterations in patterns of interaction with her partner, significant others, and in her internal and external environment are also critical attributes of consciousness in the woman's evolving pattern of pregnancy.

The experience of pregnancy has been described as a period of disequilibrium constituting a significant turning point in a woman's pattern that alters future life adjustments (Tanner, 1969). Pregnancy is often enumerated as a time of crisis in which a certain amount of psychological reorganization takes place in order to master the tasks associated with the crisis and reach a new developmental stage or a higher level of consciousness (Leifer, 1977; Rubin, 1976).

Leifer (1977) found that the most significant developmental task of pregnancy was the acceptance and emotional incorporation of the unborn child. The significance of this attachment process lies in the reorganization of a woman's life and the integration of another pattern within her own unitary pattern. Gara and Tilden (1984) introduced the concept of "adjusted control" in their qualitative research conducted with pregnant women. By "adjusted control," the authors referred to those women who viewed their pregnancies as positive and had achieved a feeling of control by accepting and coming to terms with their pregnancies through a process of psychological reorganization.

Clearly, the literature suggests and research findings support that the experience of pregnancy is characterized by a change in a woman's perceptions of movement, time, space, and consciousness. In pregnancy and in childbirth, alterations in the pregnant woman's perceptions will lead to a change in the function and structure of her pattern. When these alterations become stabilized by the exchange of energy in the pregnant woman's interaction with the environment, a new order emerges at a higher level of consciousness. For the pregnant woman, this may occur in the experience of high risk pregnancy or in the birthing process itself.

MANIFESTATIONS OF PATTERN IN PREGNANCY DURING HOSPITALIZATION

The experience of hospitalization superimposes additional alterations on the pregnant woman's perception both of her pattern and of person-environment interactions. Again, this assessment framework for the emerging pattern of health may be seen from the manifestations of movement, space, time, and consciousness.

Women who are hospitalized for the management of high risk pregnancy are "therapeutically" confined. Movement is restricted to bed or within the room, nursing unit, or hospital. This confinement is in addition to the confinement implicit in the alteration of movement during the experience of pregnancy. A woman's pattern of movement also may be limited by the length of intravenous tubing. If electronic fetal monitoring is required to assess the well-being of the fetus and/or the woman's pattern of uterine activity and contractions, monitoring belts may also restrict her movement and confine her to bed rest. Her movement patterns are iatrogenically restricted to the length of the intravenous tubing, the cord that plugs in the intravenous infusion pump, and the cords that attach the ultrasonic Doppler and tocotransducer to the electronic fetal monitor.

When hospitalized, time becomes routinized according to hospital schedules: when vital signs are taken, when meals are served, when nursing shifts begin and end, when visitors are permitted, when bathing is performed, and when "morning care" is done. Inevitably, hospitalization disrupts the pregnant woman's normal routine and pattern. The perception that time moves more slowly is consistently associated with the decreased movement imposed by therapeutic bed rest. The celebrations and rites of passage experienced by pregnant women, such as wearing maternity clothes, having baby showers, preparing the baby's room, and attending childbirth preparation classes, are frequently put on hold with the uncertainty of a high risk pregnancy. Progression through the tasks of pregnancy may be interrupted or suspended, by the experience of hospitalization for the management of a complicated pregnancy.

Confined in an unfamiliar environment, separated from her partner, family, friends, work, and colleagues, a woman's perception of space is limited to what can be seen from the bed, the room, the length of the intravenous tubing. The viewpoint of always being in a reclining or sitting position also alters a woman's visual field and perception of space, further altering her pattern. The shared space and lack of privacy are further alterations which may be disruptive to a woman's pattern. Indeed, even sleeping in a twin bed may be problematic for women who are accustomed to sleeping with their partners in a larger space. The whole notion of living and experiencing an important part of one's life from the confines of a hospital bed is troubling for most women and may precipitate additional stressors associated with the lack of control implicit in hospitalization.

The pregnant woman's normal pattern of interactions and relationships with others is also altered and changed by the disruptions associated with hospitalization. She spends more time alone or with individuals she is not used to interacting with (for example, her roommate, nurses, and physicians). The focus of her consciousness is shifted abruptly to self and to the unborn child's well-being.

Newman (1986) describes her awareness of what restricted movement means in terms of time, space, and the expansion of consciousness. She states: "The freedom to come and go as one pleases, when one pleases, is taken for granted until circumstances render that movement impossible or unwise. The restriction of movement forces one into a realm beyond space and time. The old ways of living and relating don't work anymore. One is confronted with one's own inner resources, the quality of one's relationships, and one's ability to live in the present."

The experience of hospitalization forces the pregnant woman into a realm beyond space and time, into new patterns of living and relating. As Newman asserts, "the developmental task is to allow the transformation of ourselves to occur as we move beyond space and time to a higher level of consciousness." For women hospitalized during the experience of high risk pregnancy, the developmental task is the same.

THE MANAGEMENT OF PRETERM LABOR

Women who are hospitalized for the management of preterm labor are confined for the management of symptoms and control of uterine activity and contractions. Preterm labor is defined as labor occurring prior to the completion of 36 weeks of gestation and is the predominant cause of preterm birth. Preterm births, although they represent only 8 to 10 percent of infants born in the United States, account for over 60 to 75 percent of the perinatal morbidity and mortality. The goal, therefore, for the management of preterm labor is to prevent further cervical dilation which may result in preterm birth and delivery of a premature infant. Comparing the interventions commonly prescribed in the management of preterm labor under the "old" paradigm and the "new" paradigm will provide a useful way to examine the application of Newman's theory of health in nursing practice.

Under the "old" paradigm the protocol used for therapeutic medical and nursing interventions in preterm labor typically includes the following practices:

- prolonged hospitalization on a high risk labor and birthing unit for observation, assessment, and electronic monitoring of uterine contractions and fetal activity;
- therapeutic bed rest: either complete bed rest, commode, shower, and/or bathroom "privileges" (again, please note the use of language to suggest the power of the health care provider in restricting a woman's pattern of movement);
- electronic fetal and uterine monitoring (this is the application of ultrasonic devices and electronic transducers for the assessment of fetal well-being and quantification of uterine activity and contractions); and
- administration of intravenous medications for tocolysis (these medications are usually referred to as tocolytics, literally meaning "to stop the uterus").

Unfortunately, the pharmacologic actions of tocolytic medications are not specific to only the uterine muscle. The actions of these drugs are systemic, uncomfortable, and potentially toxic, causing adverse side effects for the pregnant woman as well as the unborn child. Magnesium sulfate, for example, is a central nervous system depressant that is widely used in the management of preterm labor. This medication literally numbs women during their experience of pregnancy and may prevent them from actively participating in decision making and caring for themselves (and their unborn babies) during hospitalization. **Magnesium** sulfate also causes significant and generalized muscle weakness (described by women as feeling limp all over), headaches, blurred vision, nausea, vomiting, decreased gastrointestinal motility (which is already decreased in pregnancy), and decreased fetal activity and reactivity.

These management strategies prescribed for the control and suppression of uterine activity for preterm labor are compatible with an "old" paradigm worldview. They focus on controlling uterine activity and contractions (symptom control); the technological monitoring and management of symptoms; finding out what is wrong (diagnosing it) and fixing it; identifying the objective causes of preterm labor (causal model); quantification of contractions with the use of electronic uterine monitoring devices; predicting; and being oriented to a view of preterm labor as a disease and/or illness to be eradicated.

It is interesting to note that even the use of risk assessment tools for the prediction of preterm labor are based on a causal, disease oriented model. These assessment tools are predictive only about 40 percent of the time. More than one half of all preterm labor cannot be predicted.

Newman's theory of health provides another perspective that radically transforms the "management" of preterm labor. This new paradigm challenges our previous notions regarding our roles as health care providers and our relationships with clients. Indeed, in this new paradigm of health, our primary intervention becomes pattern recognition. The effectiveness of this intervention is evaluated in the empowerment of pregnant women to actively participate in the assessment and recognition of their own patterns.

Newman's theory of health as expanding consciousness emanates from this notion of pattern recognition. Indeed, Newman claims that nursing's primary intervention is pattern recognition. Pattern recognition is one of the essential attributes in the new paradigm of health, which has even been referred to as the "paradigm of pattern." This emerging paradigm is typically characterized as relational, patterned, acausal, probabilistic, unitary, intuitive, qualitative, individualistic, subjective, and innovative. The paradigm of health as pattern does not disregard or eliminate the traditional view of health. Rather, this new paradigm incorporates the characteristics of the old paradigm fully into its own, evolving a new explication of wholeness and consciousness.

A holistic approach to preterm labor in this new paradigm of health might consider a woman's internal stress, social support network, and general health as potential aspects of the underlying pattern shown in the increased uterine activity and contractions of preterm labor. Lewis Mehl, an obstetrician and practitioner of holistic medicine, identified four characteristics that he believed were manifested in the experience of preterm labor: (1) lack of social support for maintaining the pregnancy, (2) significant stress perceived among family members where women unconsciously saw an early delivery as a solution to family problems, (3) limited ability to deal with pressures around them and the tendency to deal with stress by avoidance, and (4) presence of health problems such as allergies and vague aches and pains where the learned response was reinforcement for illness (Peterson & Mehl, 1984). Women learned that they received attention when ill and none when they were healthy (Goer, 1987). Each of these characteristics suggests a pattern that is part of the woman's underlying life process, a pattern of the whole, which may be expressed in pregnancy as an adverse physiological manifestation such as preterm labor.

In Mehl's holistic identification of contributing factors to the characteristics manifested as uterine contractions, he poses a phenomenologically based prenatal screening tool utilized by existentially oriented clinicians (Grimes, Mehl, McRae, & Peterson, 1983). Unlike other systems in which the individual is scored on various factors considered potential risks in all pregnancies, this screening tool considers each woman individually in the totality of her own pattern. This holistic approach and implementing of a phenomenological risk screening tool for pregnancy and childbirth, are consistent with the new paradigm of health, which asserts that pregnancy and birth complications are not merely explications of random, physiological phenomena, but expressions of the total pattern of the person in interaction with her environment.

Herein lies the relationship of the nurse and client as partners and active participants in this new paradigm of health. By assisting the woman experiencing preterm labor (or any other complication of pregnancy) in the identification and clarification of her life pattern, the nurse affirms and validates the woman's ability to integrate the experience of high risk pregnancy into her pattern of the whole. When the nurse has an opportunity to meet with the woman prior to the explication of high risk pregnancy and/or preconceptually, the nurse may guide the woman in identifying patterns in her life that may predispose her to the manifestation of a high risk complication during pregnancy. In this manner, the nurse may facilitate the woman's knowing her own pattern and assist her with identification and mediation of those behaviors or environmental characteristics that may create potential risk to herself or unborn child during pregnancy.

The woman experiencing a high risk pregnancy may experience feelings of uncertainty and fear related to the threat perceived to herself and/or her unborn child. In assessing and interacting with the pregnant woman, the nurse can—through pattern recognition—assist and participate in the client's integration of her perception of self and unborn child as a unitary whole. This process of reintegration facilitates the experience of healing that comes when the individual reestablishes a sense of balance with the universe through a change of mind, or a transformation in attitudes, values, and beliefs (Ferguson, 1980). The integration of high risk pregnancy, as an experience "to be claimed and learned from" in relationship to the pattern of the whole, becomes a critical developmental task of pregnancy. As the woman assumes the role of mother, she integrates the reality of her unborn child into her pattern. It is this pattern recognition that is the turning point in the evolution of consciousness that is health (Newman, 1986).

THE PATTERNS OF PREGNANCY

For the client and nurse, pattern recognition becomes an invaluable assessment methodology that guides nursing and delegated medical interventions. For example, the recognition of the pattern of uterine contractions in the woman experiencing preterm labor enables the client and nurse to identify possible alterations and adjustments in activity (therapeutic bed rest, commode and shower "privileges"), environmental stimuli (visitors, unfamiliar noises, nurses), physiological stimuli (full bladder, constipation, elevated temperature, leaking amniotic fluid), diet and fluid intake (hydration status), position changes (left lateral recumbent, supine), and medications (timing and dosage of tocolytics). The woman's individual pattern of uterine activity and contractions are assessed by both the client and the nurse in the management of preterm labor.

The palpation of uterine contractions by the nurse provides another means of assessing the client holistically. Certainly the frequency, duration, and intensity of the uterine contractions can be appreciated through palpation of the woman's abdomen. However, like the palpation of a pulse, the human touch becomes a means of integrating and experiencing the patterns of the client and nurse in a mutual exchange of energy. In the act of uterine palpation, the nurse is able to perceive anxiety, tension, and warmth in the pregnant woman—as well as the movement of the unborn child. Touching the client in the assessment of uterine activity and contractions enables the nurse to demonstrate presence, support, and caring for the person in the totality of her experience of high risk pregnancy.

The pattern of fetal movement, monitored by the woman to assess the well-being of her unborn child, becomes another explication of the underlying pattern of the unborn child in relationship to the mother's pattern. A knowing of the pattern within a pattern and the influence of diet, activity, and medications on her unborn child, empowers the pregnant woman to care for her unborn child. Specific tools have been developed for the assessment of fetal movement patterns by pregnant women. These tools affirm the pregnant woman's ability to get in touch with her unborn child's pattern of activity and movement and provide her health care providers with information regarding fetal well-being.

Daily fetal movement counts, or kick counts, are well documented in the obstetrical literature and research to provide pregnant women and their health care providers the *best* assurance about the health and well-being of the unborn child. This record is felt to be superior and more sensitive than most of the sophisticated fetal surveillance techniques and electronic, ultrasonic monitoring devices and equipment (and far less expensive). These daily fetal movement counts also have the advantages of promoting maternal-fetal attachment, validating a woman's knowledge about her unborn child, and empowering the pregnant woman to actively participate in her prenatal care while providing prenatal care for her child. The subtle changes in the pattern of fetal activity are usually first recognized by the mother. She is the most sensitive monitor of changes and alterations in the pattern of her unborn child's movement, changes which may indicate a change in fetal health.

Assisting the pregnant woman with identifying the pattern of her unborn child's movement is an invaluable means of getting in touch with the unborn child's pattern prior to birth. The pattern recognition of fetal movements also helps the health care provider determine the ideal time for monitoring the fetal heart rate in response to activity or uterine contractions with electronic fetal monitoring (non-stress tests and contraction stress tests). The pattern of the unborn child's heart rate in response to movement becomes an indicator of his or her neurological integrity and reactivity. The baseline, variability, and periodic changes associated with the fetal heart rate become the parameters for assessing well-being of the unborn child when evaluated over a period of time. In fact, the interpretation of the fetal heart rate strip is evaluated to be reassuring or non-reassuring on the basis of the presence and consistency of these pattern parameters, which are part of the unborn child's pattern of the whole.

The paradox that exists in the partnership of the client and nurse in the new paradigm of health can be seen in the significance of the patterns that the client and nurse come to know in their interaction. It is in understanding the whole, the "maternal-fetal unit," that both the client and nurse come to know and understand the parts better, the mother and the unborn child. Perhaps it is also a paradox that a woman has the opportunity to come to know and understand herself and her pattern (as well as the pattern of her unborn child) in the experience of high risk pregnancy. It is in the inward interaction with the self as the pattern of the whole, the movement "within" when the movement "without" is restricted, that the woman experiences her self and her unborn child in intensely intimate and insightful ways. The experience of high risk pregnancy, therefore, becomes an opportunity for knowing and understanding the self as pattern, leading to the insight that accelerates the evolution of consciousness manifested in the love of the mother for her child.

As a woman's perceptions of movement, time, space, and consciousness are altered during pregnancy (and in the management of high risk pregnancy through the prescriptions of therapeutic bed rest, hospitalization, and administration of tocolytic medications), the capacity of the pregnant woman to interact with her environment is altered. As the quantity and quality of this interaction is affected, the level of consciousness determining the client's reality is altered and expanded. In the presence of the nurse, the physical manifestations experienced by the client may be reflected back in a manner enhancing the client's ability to recognize and integrate the characteristics of her experience into her pattern of the whole. In experiencing the insight that Newman (1986) equates with pattern recognition, the client participates in the expansion of consciousness, the process of the evolution of consciousness that is the process of health. It is in the expansion of consciousness that the client, as partner and active participant in the experience of high risk pregnancy, is able to gain insight regarding her pattern and experience health.

A PATTERN-BASED PROGRAM FOR MANAGING PRETERM LABOR

Recently, a new method of administering a very low dose of a tocolytic medication was proposed by Fung Lam (1989) and Pam Gill (Gill, Smith, & McGregor, 1989) for the management of preterm labor. Their research findings described the therapeutic efficacy of this mode of tocolytic therapy that uses a small, portable, infusion device (similar to an insulin pump). This program for the management of preterm labor was based on administering subcutaneous terbutaline (a tocolytic medication) according to a woman's individual circadian pattern of uterine activity and contractions. A preterm labor log was developed by these researchers to determine the dosage schedule for the administration of subcutaneous terbutaline in the management of uterine contractions. Electronic uterine monitoring devices were used by the women participating in this program to assess their patterns of uterine activity and contractions.

A group of perinatologists and nurses at Abbott Northwestern Hospital in Minneapolis have developed a program for self-monitoring of preterm labor, which is based on the concept of pattern recognition and uses this method of tocolytic therapy. Women with preterm labor are invited to actively participate in the management of their pregnancy using this therapy. (We refer to this therapy as continuous subcutaneous terbutaline therapy.) Nurses instruct women in learning techniques for the self-palpation of their uterine activity and contractions. Women are instructed in recording this information in a diary, which is then used to develop a schedule for the administration of subcutaneous terbutaline. This written record provides a document for women to record their pattern of uterine activity and contractions; the basal rate and bolus doses of terbutaline they self-administer using the pump, their pulse rate (an indicator of their tolerance and response to the medication), their pattern of activity, as well as the pattern of their unborn child's activity and movements. Women are taught pump programming procedures for self-administration of the tocolytic medication, as well as how to insert the infusion set and change the syringe for the maintenance of this therapy. Even the pump has settings that allow the automatic administration of terbutaline according to patterns preprogrammed in the profile mode of the pump. Although this therapy is initiated in the hospital, most women are able to go home within several days and are followed by perinatal nurses with expertise in home management of high risk pregnancy. At home, these women continue to monitor their own patterns of uterine activity and self-administer terbutaline based on their self-palpation and assessment of uterine activity patterns.

This program of pattern recognition for the management of preterm labor exemplifies Newman's theory of health as expanding consciousness. This is characterized by the active participation of the pregnant woman in partnership with her health care providers in the totality of her experience of preterm labor. The client actively and knowledgeably participates in her obstetrical care (practice), in the research evaluating the effectiveness of this mode of tocolytic therapy (research), and in the development and evaluation of educational materials developed for use with this therapy (education).

This program, based on pattern recognition, is research as praxis (Newman, 1990). Characterized by negotiation, reciprocity (of data and theory, of the researcher and the researched), and empowerment, this program transforms the traditional management of preterm labor by inviting pregnant women to actively participate as partners in their own care. Through pattern recognition, these women come to know and experience their bodies in pregnancy and their pattern of the whole. This pattern is experienced in the totality of their interaction with the environment within (their pattern of uterine activity and the pattern of their unborn child) and without (the pattern of their relationships with their partner, families, and health care providers).

By operationalizing the concepts of negotiation, reciprocity, and empowerment, these women—our patients—have become our teachers. They have taught us what we need to know in order to help other women with preterm labor; they have taught their physicians, their families, and each other. These women with preterm labor are partners and participants with us in learning how to use this therapy, and in sharing and collecting data and information that will help determine which other women could benefit from participation in this pattern-based program for the management of preterm labor. This is the negotiation, reciprocity, and empowerment that Newman (1990) and Lather (1986) have described as research as praxis.

Clinical expertise in knowledgeably using this therapy and monitoring patterns of uterine activity and contractions has been shared with our clients. In our partnership with these women, we have learned and continue to learn about pattern recognition, not just as it pertains to preterm labor, but as it pertains to women's experiences in pregnancy and our own experiences as health care providers.

The most exciting part of this program is that women are able to recognize their preterm labor as part of the explicate pattern of their own unique and evolving pattern as whole individuals, as women, and as mothers. They are able to assess their pattern of uterine activity and contractions through self-palpation and respond to a change in uterine activity with administration of terbutaline. Instead of requiring prolonged hospitalization (weeks to months) for the management of preterm labor with intravenous medications and electronic uterine monitoring, these women are able to stay home, monitor their own uterine activity patterns, and administer their own tocolytic medication. This is shared management. This is empowerment. This is Newman's theory of health based upon pattern recognition in practice.

The activity level and pattern of movement in pregnant women may actually increase at home. They are typically on "couch rest" versus "bed rest," and can continue to monitor their uterine activity and contractions in response to any changes in activity while at home. Their perception of time is still altered, but the disruptions typically associated with hospitalization are minimized when surrounded by the comforts and familiarity of their own "space," in their own homes, with their partners and families. These women are empowered to know and recognize their patterns of interaction with theirselves, their bodies, and their unborn children in ways not realized prior to the diagnosis of preterm labor. The increased awareness of their own pattern of uterine activity and contractions, their body's response to the administration of subcutaneous terbutaline as basal rates and bolus doses, the pattern of their unborn child's movement, are all explications of health. The insight that is gained when the movement "within" occurs as the movement "without" is restricted, accelerates the expansion of consciousness during the pregnant woman's experience of preterm labor.

Learning to recognize environmental stimuli that may alter the pattern of uterine activity (for example, visitors, eating, certain times of day), these women come to know their own unique, circadian patterns of contractions in the totality of their pattern of the whole. This pattern recognition in the context of self in interaction with their unborn child is a unique opportunity to spend time with and learn about their unborn child. Indeed, as one pregnant woman has said: "I feel like I really know what's going on with my body. I can trust it again, and I know I am doing something very important for myself and my baby. . . ." Perhaps this is "the gift" of preterm labor.

Knowledge in this program of pattern recognition is dependent upon the assumption that the process of pattern recognition *is* the content. This means that in the open and interactive nature of the evolving pattern, the process of interacting with one's own pattern is the content (Newman, 1990). This program, which is based on pattern recognition and learning to respond to one's pattern on the basis of this recognition, results in the acquisition of knowledge " . . . in processes through which we actually make and remake ourselves as human beings" (Morgan, 1983). As Newman asserts, this reciprocity between the nurse and the woman experiencing preterm labor provides the change-enhancing context in which "the intersection between people's self-understanding and the researcher's theoretical stance" facilitates the empowerment of the participants to "understand and change their situations. This is what research on health as expanding consciousness is all about" (Newman, 1990).

BECOMING PARTNERS

Sometimes the explications of our patterns may be manifested and recognized as illness or disease. I believe preterm labor is an explication of a woman's pattern that must be honored and attended to, not merely managed or suppressed. In this pattern-based program for the management of preterm labor, the woman's experience of preterm labor is attended to and honored. This experience can be a "gift" for both the pregnant woman and the nurse in their partnership with each other.

As Newman says, we are called to ". . . embrace 'our' present situation and allow 'ourselves' to be transformed by it . . . to go beyond 'ourselves' and beyond reason into a new order of reality, a new level of consciousness" (Newman, 1986). In our own experiences as nurses practicing at this new level, we learn that "defeat, failure, and vulnerability are equally as important as success, power, and gratifying relationships" (Newman, 1986). When we claim, learn from, and embrace our life experiences, they become our vehicles to come to know and interact with the evolving patterns of other women who may experience the defeat, failure, and vulnerability frequently manifested in the experience of high risk pregnancy. This program is the gift that becomes the vehicle for women to recognize their patterns and knowledgeably participate in the experience of their preterm labor.

In Newman's (1990) article about her theory of health as praxis, she says, "A funny thing happened on the way to developing a method to examine expanding consciousness. In the process, we discovered that sharing our perceptions of the person's pattern with the person was meaningful to the participants and stimulated new insights regarding their lives. We discovered that *our* participation in the process made a difference in *our own lives.*"

This is the gift, the invitation to each of us, that Newman (1986) describes in her theory of health. Newman's theory of health as expanding consciousness is an affirmation of the gift we all share with each other in the experiences of our lives, if we choose to look for that gift and take the time to unwrap it in the unfolding of our own patterns. For truly, "every experience of life is a gift to be claimed and learned from" (Newman, 1986).

For women with preterm labor, the gift is also there for them. It may not immediately present itself, but it will be there, wrapped in the recognition of their own evolving patterns and in the nurses who assist them in the process of that pattern recognition. It will be there in the love and support of their family and friends, and in the birth of their baby. Yes, that is the gift.

As nurses, we become partners and participants in expanding consciousness through the processes of research and knowledge development inherent in our practice and in our interaction with clients and other health professionals. As partners in caring, nurses have the unique opportunity to share the gifts of their experiences to assist clients and other health professionals in claiming and learning from the experiences of their own lives, the gifts that are manifest in their own patterns.

Becoming partners in the new paradigm of health, the paradigm of pattern, necessitates a partnership that is based on a holistic view which is relational and oriented in the process of becoming, of evolving and expanding consciousness, and of health. To empower nurses to engage in mutuality with clients and collegiality with other health professionals also means becoming partners with ourselves. As Newman asserts: "Becoming partners with clients and other health professionals means becoming partners ourselves" (1986).

The gift we give to others as nurses through the experience of pattern recognition is the essence and the purpose of our practice in the new paradigm. For it is in giving the gift of ourselves, that we come to know and understand ourselves. As we become partners in health with our clients and colleagues, our patterns become one, and the gifts we give to each other become the gifts we give to ourselves.

ACKNOWLEDGEMENTS

The opportunity to share my experience using Newman's theory of health as expanding consciousness has truly been a gift for me. I would like to thank Margaret Newman for sharing her theory of health with me and helping me to see my own pattern unfolding and evolving as a doctoral student in nursing. Her invitation to present this application of her theory in practice with her in Miami was an extraordinary gift to me, and I am sincerely thankful. My colleagues at work have been a source of encouragement and support to me, both in my returning to academic study, and in the continuing development of this program of pattern recognition for the management of preterm labor. The women who have participated in this program have truly been my teachers. It is to them, too, that I express my sincere appreciation. It has truly been a privilege to participate in this process of expanding consciousness with each of you. Thank you, for sharing your gifts with me.

REFERENCES

Ferguson, M. (1980). *The aquarian conspiracy: Personal and social transformation in the 1980's.* Los Angeles: J. P. Tarcher.

Gara, E. O., & Tilden, V. P. (1984). Adjusted control: An explanation for women's positive perceptions of their pregnancies. *Health Care for Women International, 5,* 427–436.

Gill, P., Smith, M., & McGregor, C. (1989). Terbutaline by pump to prevent recurrent preterm labor. *The American Journal of Maternal Child Nursing, 14*(3), 163–167.

Goer, H. (1987, fall). Holistic approach to preterm labor. *Childbirth Educator, 8.*

Grimes, L., Mehl, L. E., McRae, J., & Peterson, G. (1983). Phenomenological risk-screening for childbirth: Successful prospective differentiation of risk for medically low-risk mothers. *Journal of Nurse-Midwifery, 28*(5), 27–30.

Lam, F. (1989). Miniature pump infusion of terbutaline—An option in preterm labor. *Contemporary OB/GYN, 33,* 52–70.

Lather, P. (1986). Research as praxis. *Harvard Educational Review, 56*(3), 257–277.

Leifer, M. (1977). Psychological changes accompanying pregnancy and motherhood. *Genetic Psychology Monographs, 95,* 55–96.

Morgan, G. (1983). Toward a more reflective social science. In G. Morgan (Ed.). *Beyond method: Strategies for social research* (pp. 368–376). Beverly Hills: Sage.

Newman, M. A. (1984). Nursing diagnosis: Looking at the whole. *American Journal of Nursing, 84,* 1496–1499.

Newman, M. A. (1986). *Health as expanding consciousness.* St. Louis: C. V. Mosby.

Newman, M. A. (1990, spring). Newman's theory of health as praxis. *Nursing Science Quarterly,* 37–41.

Peterson, G. H., & Mehl, L. (1984). *Pregnancy as healing.* Berkeley, CA: Mindbody Press.

Rubin, R. (1976). Maternal tasks in pregnancy. *Journal of Advanced Nursing, 1,* 367–376.

Tanner, L. (1969). Developmental tasks of pregnancy. In B. Bergersen (Ed.). *Current Concepts in Clinical Nursing,* pp. 292–297. St. Louis: C. V. Mosby.

Part 7

Levine's Conservation Model

15

Conservation and Integrity

Myra E. Levine

For two decades, nurses have been assured that the proper practice of nursing depends upon the identification of nursing theory. Indeed, some nursing authors look with disdain at the pre-theory state of the art, proclaiming it "untheoretical" (Meleis, 1985) and thereby unacceptable to the enlightened. In the past 20 years there have been countless workshops, seminars, and conferences describing the essential role that theory must play in nursing practice. The letter of invitation to this conference said:

> The goal . . . is to bring nursing theorists and conceptual frameworks closer to the practicing nurse . . . to introduce the subject to those nurses who have not been exposed to it before, and to assist those nurses who are familiar with conceptual models to apply them in a practical way in their clinical practice (Gardner, 1989).

So, in still another conference, the effort to build the bridge between the theorist and the practitioner is at hand. While the literature on theory grows, the response of the practicing nurse has been a voiceless refusal—not out of ineptitude or ignorance but rather because the workplace insists on its own priorities.

There is little time to do what must be done—and little left for experimentation. It is not that the practicing nurse hasn't tried. A recent advertisement in the *Toronto Globe and Mail* (Feb. 10, 1990) seeks:

> Clinical Nurse Specialist
> Nursing Conceptual Frameworks
>
> This is an 18–24 month term position during which the successful applicant will lead the Nursing Division from theory to practice in the implementation of a new Conceptual Framework. The position will focus on implementing theory into practice . . . . A knowledge of Nursing Conceptual Frameworks (R.O.Y. and/or O.R.E.M.) [sic] and an appreciation of the current issues of nursing practice are essential.

Nurses want to understand and use theory. The theorists quote Kaplan (1954): "Theory is of practice and must stand or fall with its practicality." For the theorist to be heeded, and the practicing nurse to use theory, there must first be a common bond of understanding between them. They need to speak the same language. The introduction of terms by the theorist that are not and have never been part of the language of the workplace invites confusion. To reject the language of practice—most notably the pathophysiological and technological terms that define the activities of practice—reinforces the distance between theorist and nurse.

The practicing nurse has a right to know exactly what the use of the conceptual model will offer both nurse and patient. However, what the theorist really believes may not be self-evident. Much of the bibliography on conceptual models has been created by self-appointed critics and interpreters. In a recent issue of *Nursing Outlook,* an updated list of current nursing literature gave six references for nursing theory, all of them collections by commentators or critics (Brandon & Hill, 1990). The self-appointed critics engage in questionable scholarship when they use each other as sources. They create a bibliography virus, but unlike its counterpart, the computer virus, it is nearly impossible to expunge. Instead, it clings to issues of translating theory into practice, using the flawed, imperfect versions that critics have created. There is a warning here that any nurse who is truly determined to understand nursing theory can achieve it best by reading the primary sources—the theorist's own words. There is no guarantee that such an enterprise will bring light and clarity, but a personal error of interpretation has the advantage, at least, of being an honest mistake (Levine, 1990).

Sometimes the mysterious language of a theory is a hint that the reader should look closely at the scientific discipline from which it is drawn. Very rarely does the critic question the concepts upon which the theory is founded, and while theorists often invoke the names of important contributors, there is no testimony to insure the accurate use of their ideas. Then there are the purists, who claim they have no debt to another discipline, but have created a pristine nursing theory that is free of all contaminants. The proponents of this strange view offer no mercy to those whom they accuse of borrowing from other disciplines (Kim, 1983; Meleis, 1985; Fitzpatrick & Whall, 1983). A recent article describes the alleged pitfalls of borrowing:

> . . . to push from within is viewed as essential for developing nursing science. . . . using frameworks from other disciplines enlarges the knowledge base of that discipline, which is a contribution to science but not to nursing science . . . . Using frameworks from other disciplines to guide practice and research is viewed as borrowing. Borrowing requires returning; the borrower returns the fruits of the knowledge development to the discipline from which it is borrowed. The most commonly borrowed frameworks come from physiology, psychology, sociology, and education (Smith, 1990).

It is naive to suggest that any discipline *owns* its knowledge, and that there is some foolish competition between disciplines that forbids the use of concepts and facts lest one be forced to return them—like a cup of sugar to an obliging neighbor. Is there a practicing nurse who believes that safe, effective care can be provided without a firm grasp of physiology, psychology, sociology, and education—or indeed, microbiology, biochemistry, history, anthropology, and mathematics? Nursing would be bereft without these vital *adjuncts* to knowledge—not borrowed, but shared in common enterprise. To shrug away the importance of the adjunctive disciplines opens the gate for the purveyors of pseudoscience, those seeking alternative and paranormal explanations. There are too many questions to be answered in nursing to dismiss the knowledge that can be tested in favor of that which must be accepted on faith (Levine, 1988).

ENERGY CONSERVATION: A UNIVERSAL CONCEPT

Conservation is a universal concept. Every elementary physics text will verify that the conservation of energy is a natural law that governs everything in the universe—living and inanimate. Feynman (1965) describes the Great Conservation Principles as "great general principles which all laws seem to follow." Conservation describes the way complex systems are able to continue to function even when severely challenged. They sustain themselves, not only in the face of immediate disruptive threats, but in such a way as to assure the vitality of future responses. This work is accomplished in the most economic way possible. A good illustration of this practice of conservation can be seen in the way a thermostat maintains the ambient temperature in a room. When the temperature of the room is the same as that set on the thermostat, nothing happens. When the temperature of the room falls, the thermostat turns on the heating system—using energy—but only until the room temperature once more reaches the specified level. It then turns itself off, rests, and is quiet. The thermostat conserves energy —uses it in the most frugal, economic, and energy-sparing fashion.

This same process of conservation is characteristic of the way that physiological functions are regulated in the body. Negative feedback is activated when something needs to be adjusted, but is quiescent otherwise. Conservation defends the wholeness of living systems by ensuring their ability to confront change appropriately and retain their unique identity. Living systems, however, are not self-sustaining. They need a constant selection of renewing nourishment from the environment. They are open systems, incessantly interacting with the environment that provides the energy and information necessary for well-being and survival.

The environment is not always "user-friendly." Successful engagement with the environment depends upon the individual's repertoire—that store of adaptations which is either built into the genes or achieved through life experience. While there are redundant or back-up systems that offer options when the initial response is insufficient, health and safety are products of a competent conservation process. The goal of conservation is health (Levine, 1967, 1973, 1989, 1990).

INTEGRITY AS HEALTH

Health has proved to be an elusive concept, defined in long paragraphs encompassing every aspect of the life span. The word health and the word whole come from the same root word. The word whole has another twin word: integrity. No one needs to be instructed in what it means to be whole, to have one's integrity respected and valued. The growth and development of every human being is the evolution of a sense of oneness—from the infant in the crib (Piaget & Inhelder, 1967), who learns there is an "in here" and an "out there," to the adult who defines his or her personal boundaries and asks to be recognized as unique. Integrity means being in control of one's life. Integrity is having the freedom to choose: to move without constraint, as slowly or as swiftly as desired, and to exercise decisions on all matters—trivial and otherwise—without apology, indebtedness, or guilt. Integrity is the experience of life, the sensations of the body and its limbs, the sensory recording of every place and time on the mind and in the spirit.

The child learns to trust the integrity of his or her body, to test it, experience it, and nurture that confidence which will serve throughout life. Every child learns to have certainty that he or she will heal when injured and be restored when ill. Everyone establishes that covenant of faith. This covenant gives strength and courage in the face of danger. The body anticipates disaster and prepares for difficulty. Wounds are promptly sealed. The course of healing can be predicted. Cells race to their specific tasks; tissues re-form themselves. The immune system learns to recognize friend and foe, self and non-self—thus protecting the body from invasion, insult, and disease. The conservation of energy protects functional integrity, but structural integrity of the body is defended by the body's talent to restore continuity and form—replicating damaged cells and making whole that which was disrupted. This is the process called healing.

Residing in the physical limits of the body, there is a self that is defined, defended, and described only by the soul that owns it. That private self is unique and whole. A person can share mere fragments of it with others. Relationships are built on scraps and pieces, imperfectly shared, even in the most intimate exchanges. Strangers are held at bay in the most mundane situations. On crowded trains and buses there is no eye contact; each person pressed against another creates space by staring into infinity. This aloofness is fiercely defended in all public places where the individual cannot gauge friend or foe and conserves energy and involvement by identifying neither. The private self knows its own secrets and cannot freely share them. The private self is the essence of selfhood, the repository of identity. The self is always wary, demanding respect at least and recognition at best. Kurt Goldstein (1963) noted that even severely brain-damaged soldiers retained, however altered, knowledge of a self. Awareness of the self is a testimony of wholeness. This awareness of a self is called independence.

Selfhood grows with the child; much of it is taught. Such learning begins in infancy, when each time the baby is awake and alert signals the beginning of an exchange between parent and infant, and the baby learns to remember a voice and recognize a face. The family is the bulwark that allows the self to form—protecting, guiding, and correcting in order to permit the child to lead a competent, self-directed life. Even that which is so guarded and private is influenced by other lives, which give meaning and value to the individual, as the individual reflects the meaning and values of the larger life of the family. Ethnicity is taught in the family, as is religious commitment. The language of the household and that of the wider world is learned in the family. In the family, the child learns of community and how to behave in those social environments particular to the child. The child learns how to behave with peers, in school, and with authority figures. As the child grows, he or she learns there are other values, which must be wed to what the family has demanded. The child must learn about the obligations of one human being to another, the limits of law, the life choices that direct education, career, and economic well-being. This process is called living.

THE CONSERVATION PRINCIPLES AS A FRAMEWORK

I have described energy conservation and the wholeness embodied in the integrity of structure, person, and society in broad terms in order to emphasize that the Conservation Principles are *not* limited only to the care of the sick in the hospital. I have borne the burden of that naive and foolish criticism for several years—ever since two misinformed graduate students wrote a chapter in which they made clear they knew more about what was in my mind than I did (Esposito & Leonard, 1980). They chose my textbook of medical-surgical nursing, *Introduction to Clinical Nursing* (Levine, 1969, 1973) as the text from which to critique my work. That text—each edition of which was named "Best Book of the Year" by the American Journal of Nursing—was begun in 1963. I was not writing a nursing theory. I was teaching medical-surgical nursing to students whose practice was in a hospital. That is the way it was in the early 60s. Even university students learned nursing in acute care institutions. The battle-cry then was "back to the bedside." Nevertheless, it was the eve of the greatest technological change in the history of health care—Pasteur, Koch, and Virchow notwithstanding.

Stephen Jay Gould said, "The mark of any good theory is that it makes coordinated sense of a string of observations otherwise independent and inexplicable" (1980). The Conservation Principles are broad generalizations designed to gather "independent and inexplicable" (Gould, 1980) concepts into an organizing framework within which nursing practice in every environment can be anticipated, predicted, and performed. In acute care institutions, nursing homes, clinics, and community health programs and in their management and administration—everywhere nursing is essential—the rules of conservation and integrity hold. The essence of specialized practice, those essential concepts that make "coordinated sense" (Gould, 1980) of the nursing act, draws its strength from the variety of options available. The use of concepts from adjunctive disciplines brings coherence to nursing problems, encouraging freedom of exploration in practice, research, and teaching without losing sight of the integrity of either the practitioner or the patient. It does so for the healthy *and* the sick. What is being conserved, if it is not health?

Yet, there is no task more complex than the provision of health care. Seeking the broad generalizations that will bring together that "string of observations" (Gould, 1980) can succeed only if bold assumptions are made, but these assumptions cannot be uninformed. Living things of every kind share the earth, and the multitude of environmental habitats exist in a vital, changing harmony. To understand the individual, the place and time of his or her living must also be understood. The physiological responses of the human body are designed to meet the constantly changing environment. Cannon (1953) described the fight or flight response of the autonomic nervous system as an effective, but primitive preparation for the individual to confront a threat. The inflammatory process and the reaction of the immune system offer a second level of protection. Selye's (1956) stress theories describe yet another form of protection from the hazards of living. Gibson (1966) describes the "perceptual systems"—the ways in which individuals gather meaningful information from the environment and thus move through it in safety. Gibson emphasizes the active involvement of the individual, writing that we do not merely see with the sensory organs of sight—we look; we do not merely hear—we listen. I have proudly cited Dubos, Selye, Gibson, and Erikson as contributing important adjunctive concepts useful for the practicing nurse. I am embarrassed by theory critics who credit me for these concepts without attribution to the proper authors (Meleis, 1985).

Individual life experiences teach how intimately the individual and the environment interact. The environment is not a backdrop on a stage, where life events are acted. Bates (1967) spoke of the "operational environment," where undetected natural forces impinge on the individual. He described all of the environment that is recorded on the sensory organs as the "perceptual environment," and the influence of language, culture, ideas, and cognition as the "conceptual environment." Categorizing the environment, however, does not make it less difficult to describe. Erikson (1969, 1975) wrote of Martin Luther and Gandhi to show how the environment is a crucial influence on the development and life purpose of the individual.

The individual cannot be understood outside of the context of a place and time. The individual cannot be separated from the influence of everything that is happening around him or her, nor indeed, from all those events—remembered and forgotten—which have created the individual as he or she is at this precise moment. Nursing can succeed only when it recognizes that the person is not summarized by the immediate present, but is burdened by a lifetime of experience—recorded not only on the tissues of the body, but on the spirit and mind as well.

The Conservation Principles were born in nursing practice. Energy conservation has always been an empiric presence in nursing care. The most basic procedures were designed to minimize the cost to the patient of activities that would be overtaxing. The directions in the procedure manuals of the 30s and 40s were marvels of conserved activity—step-by-step instructions designed to complete tasks in the most expeditious ways possible.

Nurses developing sophisticated research protocols are proving once again how essential conservation of energy is in patient care. The suspicion that less energy was used when the cardiac patient was allowed to use a commode or the bathroom, or bathe in the shower rather than in bed (Winslow, 1982), has been substantiated by studies that used physiological parameters to measure demand on the patient's heart. Intensive therapies that make extraordinary demands of patients demonstrate how the conservation of energy is not simply preventing tiredness. Fatigue has new meaning for those who have had extended radiation or chemotherapy. The displacement of energy to the defense of assaulted cells leaves the individual without the strength for ordinary activities. Even walking—lifting one foot after the other—becomes a momentous task. Unusual events that test the conservation of energy to its limits demonstrate how nursing interventions—scaled to the individual's ability—are dependent upon providing care that makes the least additional demand possible.

The practice of conservation in nursing is dedicated to providing the best possible health status available to the individual. To begin with the right genes and a social environment that permits healthy choices are major advantages. The health care system, however, cannot restrict itself to only those who possess such advantages, nor can it prescribe approved life-styles while scorning those it believes harmful. The practice of true prevention in our society is hindered by two questionable viewpoints. First is the widespread notion that stress is the cause of all disease, and that its effects can be eliminated if only the individual wills it. The second viewpoint, arising from the first, says that sick people have only themselves to blame for their illnesses (Ryan, 1976). This strange distortion of reality trivializes crucial issues. Moral censure rests on those who do not exercise regularly and eat fast-food hamburgers for lunch. The introduction of oat bran into cereals and the removal of tropical oils from cookies is an imperfect kind of prevention.

A true preventive measure, such as eliminating smoking, is thwarted by claims of privacy and the political clout of the subsidized tobacco growers. Prevention is an issue of social integrity. The fatal measles cases throughout the nation are testimony of the failure to maintain the immunization program that almost wiped out the disease five years ago. True preventive measures would not permit one of the highest infant death rates in the world. A society that truly cared about prevention would provide access to health care, safe food and shelter, decent schooling, and economic stability for all. The cholesterol wars belong in the research laboratories, not on the grocer's shelf. Cancer death rates have hardly budged, despite improved diagnosis, therapies, and a consciousness of the dangers of a polluted environment. Overwhelming health problems are hardly addressed, and programs dealing with drug abuse and the spread of HIV retrovirus are seriously underfunded. Infants are now dying from these twin plagues. Unhappily, the shortage of nurses now—at a time when more nurses are practicing than ever before—is a shortage of the highly skilled nurses who can function in critical care units. There is a costly sacrifice every time an individual enters the health care system. Whether in an intensive care unit or a weight management class, the individual gives up a measure of personal independence and freedom by entering the health care system. The labeling of persons as clients reinforces that dependency because a client is a follower. The provenance of the word patient is sufferer. It is the condition of suffering that makes it possible to set independence aside and accept the services of another person. It is the challenge of the nurse to provide the individual with appropriate care without losing sight of the individual's integrity, to honor the trust that the patient has placed in the nurse, and to encourage the participation of the individual in his or her own welfare. The patient comes in trust and dependence only for as long as the services of the nurse are needed. The nurse's goal is always to impart knowledge and strength so that the individual can resume a private life—no longer a patient, no longer dependent. I want the patient to walk away from me as an independent individual.

CONCLUSION

There are four Conservation Principles, and they have implications for every nursing situation. They function as a unity, concerned with the integrity of the whole person, but, nevertheless, they permit individual examination of specific nursing problems. Focusing on one principle is useful and productive for research purposes, when the proposal must be finely honed in order to find an appropriate methodology. However, when it is a person who is being studied, there should be a focus on the wholeness of that person. Every patient displays some problems in each of the areas the Conservation Principles describe. Concerns for energy conservation and structural, personal, and social integrity are always present—though one area may present a more demanding problem than another. These areas can be explored individually, but they cannot be separated from the person. The use of the commode for the cardiac patient is measurable in the language of energy conservation, but the elements of privacy and social restraint can hardly be ignored by the nurse. The social integrity of the homeless is utterly disrupted, but the humane issues must be addressed by nursing.

Emphasizing the integrity of the patient brings integrity to the nursing profession and the individual nurse. Bringing together the best science and the most devoted humanism is the ultimate aim of nursing. In finding, valuing, and cherishing the integrity of the patient, the nurse's integrity is acknowledged and rewarded.

REFERENCES

Bates, M. (1967, February). Naturalist at large. *Natural History, 76,* 12–16.

Brandon, A. N., & Hill, D. R. (1990). Selected list of nursing books and journals. *Nursing Outlook, 38* (2), 86–97.

Cannon, W. B. (1953). *Bodily changes in pain, hunger, fear and rage.* New York: Harper Torchbooks.

Dubos, R. (1965). *Man Adapting.* New Haven: Yale University Press.

Esposito, C. E., & Leonard, M. K. (1980). Myra Estrin Levine. In J. George (Ed.). *Nursing theories: The base for professional nursing practice* (pp. 150–163). Englewood Cliffs, NJ: Prentice-Hall.

Erikson, E. (1969). *Gandhi's truth.* New York: W.W. Norton.

Erikson, E. (1975). *Life history and the historical moment.* New York: W.W. Norton.

Feynman, R. (1965). *The character of physical law.* Cambridge, MA: MIT Press.

Fitzpatrick, J., & Whall, A. (1983). *Conceptual models for nursing: Analysis and application.* Bowie, MD.: Robert J. Brady.

Gibson, J. E. (1966). *The senses considered as perceptual systems.* Boston: Houghton-Mifflin.

Gould, S. J. (1980). This view of life: The belt of an asteroid. *Natural History, 89,* 26–33.

Goldstein, K. (1963). *Human nature.* New York: Schocken.

Kaplan, A. (1954). *The conduct of inquiry.* Scranton, PA.: Chandler.

Kim, H. S. (1983). *The nature of theoretical thinking in nursing.* Norwalk, CT: Appleton-Century-Crofts.

Levine, M. E. (1967). The four conservation principles of nursing. *Nursing Forum.* 6 (1), 45–49.

Levine, M. E. (1969). *Introduction to clinical nursing.* Philadelphia: F. A. Davis.

Levine, M. E. (1973). *Introduction to clinical nursing* (2nd Ed.). Philadelphia: F. A. Davis.

Levine M. E. (1988). Antecedents from adjunctive disciplines: Creation of nursing theory. *Nursing Science Quarterly. I* (1), 16–21.

Levine, M. E. (1989). The conservation principles twenty years later. In J. Riehl-Sisca (Ed.). *Conceptual models for nursing practice* (pp. 325–337). Norwalk, CT: Appleton-Century-Crofts.

Levine, M. E. (1990 February-March) *Theorism and the theorists.* Paper presented at the University of Alberta and the University of Illinois at Chicago.

Meleis, A. (1985). *Theoretical nursing: Development and progress.* Philadelphia: J. B. Lippincott.

Piaget, J., & Inhelder, B. (1967). *The child's conception of space.* New York: W. W. Norton.

Ryan, W. (1976). *Blaming the victim.* New York: Vintage.

Selye, H. (1956). *The stress of life.* New York: McGraw-Hill.

Smith, M. J. (1990). Knowledge development: Pushing from within or pulling from without. *Nursing Science Quarterly, 2* (4), 156.

16

Application of Levine's Conservation Model to Nursing the Homeless Community

Jane B. Pond

OVERVIEW OF COMMUNITY HEALTH NURSING

Community health nursing practice is aimed at maximizing the health and well-being of populations at risk. It recognizes the "complexities of persons and their environments" and values "knowledge-based practices for the prevention of illness and the promotion of health" (Hanchett, 1988).

Community health nursing, as defined by the American Nurses' Association Conceptual Model of Community Health Nursing, focuses on the consideration that health is influenced by many factors found within people and their environments. "The dominant responsibility is to the population as a whole" (American Nurses' Association, 1980).

Community health nurses provide direct patient care in clinics, homes, and other creative settings. They deal with the health of an aggregate population—identifying risk factors for illness, disability, and death. Efforts are made to collaborate with the community in planning and implementing activities designed to promote the health of the community. Conceptual models have provided the structure to design such programs.

"Conceptual models that have the greatest application to community health nursing view people as being in constant continuous interaction within their environment" (Lee & Lancaster, 1988). Community health nursing has historically emphasized aspects of epidemiology in its practice models.

Hanchett identified four nursing theorists—Orem, Roy, King, and Rogers—as providing unique perspectives on the practice of community nursing (1988). Several other theories have also been used to address the problems of the homeless community. Bowdler and Barrell (1987) used the Neuman Systems Model as a framework to assess the multivariate health needs of the homeless community in Richmond, Virginia. This framework was used to identify the intrapersonal, interpersonal, and extrapersonal stressors that create instability within the individual and thus the aggregate community. Hogue's epidemiologic framework was employed by Francis (1987) to synthesize the current literature on the "interactions among prevalent agents, powerless hosts, and a hostile environment in producing homelessness." Orem's model of self-care was used by a nurse practitioner to foster dignity and self-esteem among the homeless, thereby promoting more efficient use of services (Park, 1989). Berne, Dato, Mason, and Rafferty (1990) used Peznecker's model of poverty to define effective nursing interventions for homeless families.

It cannot be denied that the homeless are a community at risk. Community nursing practice must focus on the collective health of the homeless community as well as the health of individual members of that group.

There are various estimates of the numbers of homeless people across the nation. According to the US Department of Housing and Urban Development, at least "two million individuals were homeless, without permanent residence" in 1984. Creative efforts were designed to reach the homeless for the 1990 census, and these numbers appear to be growing. This population has been traditionally identified with the chronic skid-row alcoholics, bag ladies, and mentally ill. This picture, however, is changing.

Today, families with children comprise more than one-third of the homeless population. Most of these families are headed by unmarried minority females. Over half of the children in these families are under five years old. It is estimated that there are as many as one million homeless children in the United States. In Philadelphia, there are approximately 900 homeless families, including more than 2,200 children (Fox & Roth, 1989).

LEVINE'S CONSERVATION MODEL: IMPLICATIONS FOR THE HOMELESS COMMUNITY

Levine's Conservation Model was developed to address the "why's" of nursing activities. "Nursing is focused on man and the complexity of his relationships with his environment" (Levine, 1967). Levine's approach to nursing has been used in a variety of clinical settings and situations. Fawcett (1989) identified the operating room, critical care unit, and emergency room as some of the acute-care settings in which Levine's model has been implemented. Schaefer and Pond (in press) describe situations including the woman in labor, the confused elderly person, the burn victim, the neurologically impaired person, and the sick toddler as examples of patient predicaments. "The individual cannot be understood outside the context of his or her predicament of time and place" (Levine, 1989a). A predicament may be described as a puzzling situation. Certainly, the homeless find themselves in a very puzzling situation.

Levine's model has been criticized because it does not address nursing practice outside the hospital setting (Glass, 1989). However, Levine (1973) states that the focus of nursing intervention is on the whole person, in health and in sickness, in the hospital, clinic, or community. Indeed, Levine asserts that "we are privileged by one license to provide an important service to the community" (1988). Levine (personal communication, November 2, 1989) acknowledges that she believes that by generalizing her model for use in the aggregate homeless community, "nursing care to that population is humanized."

Levine's Conservation Model provides an effective organizing framework for the ambulatory care of the homeless (Pond, in press). The concepts of environment, health, illness, and nursing have particular relevance for community nursing practice and provide guidance to caring for the homeless community.

The three components—operational, perceptual, and conceptual—of the external environment cannot be separated from the person. The operational environment is not directly perceived by the individual. The operational environment includes radiation, microorganisms, and pollutants (Levine, 1989a). Focusing on the operational environment directs the community nurse to assess the quality of the air surrounding homeless people huddled over steam vents. The community nurse will, therefore, screen this community for exposure to the tubercle bacillus, which thrives in an undernourished, ill host living in crowded conditions.

The perceptual environment is perceived by the senses. Sounds, sensations, and odors provide information that defines a person's safety, identity and purpose (Levine, 1989a). Examination of the perceptual environment can lead the community health nurse to consider the effects of the windchill factor in developing public policies for the safety of people living on the streets.

The conceptual environment is composed of the ideas, beliefs, traditions, and judgments that influence all behavior (Levine, 1973). The individual and the community of which he or she is a part possess cultural traditions. There is camaraderie among the homeless and traditions that are as significant as those in the cultures that may have excluded these people. "The challenge for nurses is to find the community—as well as the strengths and weaknesses lodged within it" (Benner, 1990).

Illness challenges the integrity of the person, and defending health and wholeness is an appropriate nursing endeavor (Levine, in press). The homeless population is not healthy. According to Levine (1973), only a society that provides individuals with "adequate food, gainful employment, educational opportunities, and excellent medical care is one in which health, in the sense of wholeness, can be obtained." Numerous studies demonstrate the common incidence within the homeless community of health problems such as trauma, cardiovascular and pulmonary disease, infestations, contact dermatitis and skin infestations, and substance abuse and mental illness (Brickner et al., 1986; Gelberg and Linn, 1989; Lindsey, 1989).

Homeless children suffer from delayed or lack of immunizations, nutritional deficits, delayed growth and development, and frequent infectious diseases (Pond, in press). They are at risk for abuse and neglect. They may have had no health care, and their mothers may not have had proper care during pregnancy.

Because this is an ill population, "nursing cannot emphasize health maintenance at the expense of its role in the care of the sick" (Levine, 1988). "Nursing is much more than health promotion, prevention, and maintenance" (Levine, 1989b). This does not mean, however, that these concepts should be ignored. If the mentally ill homeless woman had undergone a screening mammogram, for example, she might not be dying of breast cancer today.

THE CONSERVATION PRINCIPLES APPLIED TO THE HOMELESS COMMUNITY

According to Levine, "Survival depends on the adaptive ability to use responses that cost the least to the individual in expense of effort and demand on his or her well being" (1989a). This "keeping together" function is the essence of conservation and, therefore, the essence of nursing.

"Wholeness is the universal target of selfhood, and conservation is the guardian activity that defends and protects it" (Levine, in press). The four Conservation Principles defined by Levine (1967) provide an approach for the nursing care of the individual and the community:

1. *Conservation of Energy.* Conservation of energy is the balancing of energy expenditures with energy resources. It is unrealistic to expect homeless people to keep clinic appointments at mealtime. They may have no other opportunity to eat that day.
2. *Conservation of Structural Integrity.* Structural change results in a change of function; healing restores structural integrity. Blood pressure screening may detect hypertension. Therapy may decrease end-organ damage and further sequelae.

3. *Conservation of Personal Integrity.* Self-identity and respect are paramount; illness/health care systems threaten personal integrity. Many homeless people seem resigned to being treated as nonpersons. In the clinic, they may not be afforded the same privacy and respect as others, especially if they appear not to have attended to their personal hygiene.

4. *Conservation of Social Integrity.* Social integrity is tied to the viability of the entire social system; isolation threatens social integrity. Who listens to the homeless? What church reaches out with food, yet closes in during morning worship?

These principles can be applied to community nursing in many ways. The principle of conservation of energy is illustrated in the following interventions:

- providing food preparation and nutrition programs in shelters and feeding sites;
- monitoring commercial blood bank practices;
- monitoring air and water quality in congregate areas;
- providing (reality-based) substance abuse and smoking cessation programs;
- facilitating transportation to services used by the homeless population; and
- teaching crisis intervention and assertiveness training.

The principle of conservation of structural integrity is illustrated in the following interventions:

- teaching about violence and abuse;
- developing injury prevention programs (for example, self-defense);
- providing safety programs in shelters;
- instructing workers about sanitation and infection control;
- improving access to health care services for uninsured patients;
- providing infectious disease screening (for AIDS, tuberculosis, and sexually transmitted diseases); and

- providing health screening (immunizations, hypertension, and mammography).

The principle of conservation of personal integrity is illustrated in these interventions:

- developing community awareness programs about issues of homelessness;
- providing appropriate, adequate living spaces and privacy;
- providing job readiness, employment, and educational programs; and
- teaching parenting skills.

The principle of conservation of social integrity is illustrated in these interventions:

- developing community resources (political, religious, cultural, and educational);
- improving delivery of appropriate free health care and social services;
- providing discussion groups for self-awareness, social interaction, and life skills;
- increasing access to entitlements/decreasing bureaucracy;
- providing recreational activities; and
- teaching coping patterns.

THE HOMELESS COMMUNITY IN PHILADELPHIA

Philadelphia Health Management Corporation's 1984 study, "Homelessness in Philadelphia: People, Needs, Services," identified four groups of homeless: the economically disadvantaged, the substance abusers, the chronically mentally ill, and the elderly (Fox & Roth, 1989). While there have been dramatic increases within these groups, the categories remain relevant for the 1990s. Together, these groups form the homeless community in Philadelphia.

The economically disadvantaged group includes unemployed or underemployed people. Mothers and children constitute the fastest growing segment of this group and within the general homeless population as well. These mothers are often very young women with small children, who had been living in marginal conditions before entering the shelter system. They have very fragile support systems for this overwhelming crisis.

The substance-abusing population includes the typical skid-row, white male alcoholic and the rapidly increasing numbers of individuals addicted to crack-cocaine. It is important to remember that we must help these patients deal with their addiction, whether they use drugs because they are homeless or are homeless because they use drugs.

The chronically mentally ill homeless constitute about 30 percent of the patients in the Philadelphia Health Management Corporation's Health Care for the Homeless Project. These individuals may be older and may be by-products of the deinstitutionalized state mental health system, or they may be younger people for whom the community system has failed. Some homeless are labeled "dually-diagnosed" with both mental illness and a substance abuse problem. These patients challenge both the mental health and drug and alcohol rehabilitation systems.

The elderly comprise a smaller portion of Philadelphia's homeless population. Approximately 6 percent of our patients are over the age of 65; many of them are chronically mentally ill.

There are many factors that have contributed to the increased numbers of homeless people in Philadelphia, its suburbs, and across the nation:

- lack of economic opportunities, particularly for poorly educated, poorly skilled individuals;
- lack of adequate, affordable housing;
- lack of appropriate resources for those in need (welfare "reform"); and
- lack of adequate treatment facilities and long-range rehabilitation programs for the chronically mentally ill and the substance abuser.

The Philadelphia homeless population is dominated by single individuals, while in the suburbs the family group is more prevalent. Nearly two-thirds of Philadelphia's homeless people living in shelters are single; most are males between the ages of 18 and 45. The unmarried heads of households are predominantly minority women from 18 to 30 years old.

What are the issues the homeless must face? A typical day for a mother with two children might involve the following:

- having to bathe, dress, feed her family and be out of the shelter by 8:00 A.M. even if there is no place to go;
- meeting with a case manager to obtain shelter for the next two weeks and to discuss saving a predetermined amount of her income to be placed toward future permanent housing;
- trying to obtain school and immunization records so the children can be placed in a new school;
- worrying whether her Women, Infants, and Children (WIC) supplements will reach her at her new location;
- trying to deal with an abusive partner who is not in the shelter, but who knows where she is;
- trekking to a distant laundry to do diapers—there is no money for Pampers;
- worrying about her vague chest pains and persistent cough, but knowing that without a medical card, health care and medicines may be unavailable;
- resisting that hit of crack, when it would be so easy—sex with a stranger in exchange for a few minutes of drug-induced pleasure; and
- trying to be a good mother, with no respite from the children and no quiet time for herself.

Since 1985, Philadelphia Health Management Corporation's Health Care for the Homeless Project has provided outreach health care and social services to urban and suburban homeless in a variety of settings. This outreach program provides community health nurses, nurse practitioners, physician's assistants, and social workers to assist patients not only with their immediate health care needs, but with their many other problems. Our teams regularly visit more than 45 shelters, day programs, and feeding sites in three counties.

Levine's model has provided a framework to guide our community nursing practice. The street outreach nurse conducted tuberculosis screening for 168 men residing on the city streets. This population, wary of and resistant to invasive procedures, agreed to be interviewed. Of those, 20 men were referred to the clinic because of a history or presence of symptoms that might indicate lung disease. None were found to have active tuberculosis, but one case of cancer was diagnosed and six men were treated for pneumonia. Without this health outreach, these men would not have received nursing care.

Community nurses provide infection control instructions to shelter staff and residents. With more than 300 women and children living in one building with limited bathrooms, one case of shigella can spread rapidly. By involving the City Health Department and working collaboratively, the outreach nurses can evaluate, treat, and control the infection.

Because family violence is a prevalent factor in homelessness, nurses provide counseling, group therapy, and self-defense programs. Homeless women and health professionals are currently planning a community workshop to address issues of violence and daily living.

Advocacy about nutrition and food preparation can be a delicate subject within the profit-driven shelter system. The City of Philadelphia reimburses the shelters on a daily, per capita basis. The meals may be of questionable nutritional benefit. This issue is particularly critical when the foods are inappropriate for the age of the residents. For example, formula and milk may not be supplied by the shelters because it is not considered food. It is also expensive. Fruit drink is generally considered the house beverage. This may result in the undernutrition of the residents. Advocacy by nurses at all levels of the outreach project resulted in the provision of healthier foods at some of the shelters.

These are some examples of the impact a model-based health focus can have on a community. There are many more such examples.

FUTURE DIRECTIONS

Levine's model presents a unique view of the human experience. It is a blueprint for the nursing profession to use in its practice, education, and research.

Research using Levine's model must delve further into the effects of the environment on health. Schaefer (in press) states, "the external and internal environments and social integrity are not the same." The elements of conservation of social integrity lead the nurse to advocate for changes that could affect the environment of the homeless community; for example, more stringent monitoring of shelter standards and practices. Community concepts in the community should be examined from the perspective of Levine's Conservation Model.

This model, developed more than 20 years ago, provides insight into current nursing practice. It is limited only by those who have a narrow perspective. It is exciting to find a model that articulates one's own beliefs about nursing practice. It is as if the proverbial light bulb has been illuminated.

Nursing has always been a significant force in community health. The profession is challenged to use Levine's Conservation Model to guide its practice.

REFERENCES

American Nurses Association. (1980). *A conceptual model of community health nursing practice.* Kansas City, MO: Author.

Benner, P. (1990). Commentary. *The American Journal of Nursing, 90*(4), 55.

Berne, A. S., Dato, C., Mason, D. J., & Rafferty, M. (1990). A nursing model for addressing the health needs of homeless families. *Image, 22*(1), 8–13.

Brickner, P., Scanlan, M., Conanan, B., Elvy, A., McAdam, J., Scharer, L., & Vicic, W. (1986). Homeless persons and health care. *Annals of Internal Medicine, 104,* 405–408.

Bowdler, J. E., & Barrell, L. M. (1987). Health needs of homeless persons. *Public Health Nursing, 4*(3), 135–140.

Fawcett, J. (1989). *Analysis and evaluation of conceptual models of nursing.* Philadelphia: F.A. Davis.

Fox, E. R., & Roth, L. (1989). Homeless Children: Philadelphia as a case study. *The Annals of the American Academy of Political and Social Science, 506,* 141–151.

Francis, M. B. (1987). Long-term approaches to end homelessness. *Public Health Nursing, 4*(4), 230–235.

Gelberg, L., & Linn, L. (1989). Assessing the physical health of homeless adults. *Journal of the American Medical Association, 262*(14), 1973–1979.

Glass, J. L. (1989). Levine's Theory of Nursing. In J. Riehl-Sisca (Ed.). *Conceptual Models for Nursing Practice* (3rd ed.) (pp. 339–358). New York: Appleton-Century-Crofts.

Hanchett, E. S. (1988). *Nursing and frameworks: Community as Client.* Norwalk, CT: Appleton & Lange.

Lee, G., & Lancaster, J. (1988). Conceptual models for community health nursing. In M. Stanhope & J. Lancaster (Eds.). *Community health nursing.* St. Louis: C.V. Mosby.

Levine, M. E. (1967). The four conservation principles of nursing. *Nursing Forum, 6,* 45–59.

Levine, M. E. (1973). *Introduction to clinical nursing.* Philadelphia: F.A. Davis.

Levine, M. E. (1988). Keynote address. *District 18 Newsletter,* Illinois Nurses' Association, *XXIV,* (6), 4–7.

Levine, M. E. (1989a). The conservation principles of nursing twenty years later. In J. P. Riehl-Sisca (Ed.). *Conceptual models for nursing practice* (3rd ed.) (pp. 325–348). Norwalk, CT: Appleton & Lange.

Levine, M. E. (1989b). The ethics of nursing rhetoric. *Image, 21*(1), 4–6.

Levine, M. E. (In press). The conservation principles—A model for health. In K. M. Schaefer & J. B. Pond (Eds.). *Levine's conservation model: A framework for nursing practice.* Philadelphia: F.A. Davis.

Lindsey, A. M. (1989). Health care for the homeless. *Nursing Outlook, 37*(2), 78–81.

Park, P. B. (1989). Health care for the homeless: A self-care approach. *Clinical Nurse Specialist, 3*(4), 171–174.

Pond, J. B. (In press). Ambulatory care for the homeless. In K. M. Schaefer & J. B. Pond (Eds.). *Levine's conservation model: A framework for nursing practice.* Philadelphia: F.A. Davis.

Schaefer, K. M. (In press). Creating a Legacy. In K. M. Schaefer & J. B. Pond (Eds.). *Levine's conservation model: A framework for nursing practice.* Philadelphia: F.A. Davis.

Schaefer, K. M., & Pond, J. B. (Eds.). (In press). *Levine's conservation model: A framework for nursing practice.* Philadelphia: F.A. Davis.

US Department of Housing and Urban Development. (1984). *A report to the secretary on the homeless and emergency shelters.* Washington, D.C.: Office of Policy Development and Research.

17

A Description of Fatigue Associated with Congestive Heart Failure: Use of Levine's Conservation Model

Karen Moore Schaefer

Everyone experiences fatigue. While acute fatigue may be a warning of more serious sequelae (muscle pain, viral infection, depression, stress, illness, anemia), chronic fatigue serves no purpose except to interfere with one's ability to function (Piper, 1986).

Understanding fatigue, whether acute or chronic, is significant to nursing because it is a common problem associated with most health-related disorders. Studying the phenomenon of fatigue in a variety of clinical populations may help to determine appropriate and significant nursing interventions. The purpose of this investigation was to describe the fatigue experience in patients with congestive heart failure.

Note: This author acknowledges the editorial assistance of Judith Aronson of the Research Department, The Allentown Hospital–Lehigh Valley Hospital Center, and the support of the nursing staff of 4C.

LITERATURE REVIEW

Fatigue has many causes (Reich, 1986), appears in the healthy and the ill (Bruera & MacDonald, 1988; Fields & Loveridge, 1988; Gregersen, 1988), can be acute or chronic (Kellum, 1986; Potempa et al., 1986), and can be muscle specific or generalized (Piper, 1986). From a nursing perspective, fatigue is conceptualized as the inability to continue to function in a given situation (Srivastava, 1986). It is often described as not having enough energy to do what one wants to do. The North American Nursing Diagnosis Association (NANDA) defines fatigue as "an overwhelming sustained sense of exhaustion and decreased capacity for physical and mental work" (Carroll-Johnson, 1989). Discussions of fatigue in the literature are frequently anecdotal (Gregersen, 1988). Some investigators have attempted to develop measures of fatigue, identify its significance, and describe its characteristic patterns (Aistars, 1987; Piper, 1986; Piper, Lindsey, & Dodd, 1987).

Haylock and Hart (1979) investigated fatigue experienced by 30 cancer patients undergoing localized radiation therapy. Their findings showed that fatigue scores increased significantly from the first to the last day of treatment, that fatigue was reduced on Sundays, and that the greatest change in fatigue scores occurred in patients undergoing the longest treatment. Sixteen major symptoms, both physiological and psychological, were associated with the fatigue experience. The symptoms that were significantly related to fatigue (tired body, tired legs, heavy load, eye strain) supported a physical rather than a psychological etiology of this phenomenon.

McCorkle (1981) conducted a study of 61 newly diagnosed lung cancer patients and 52 multiple sclerosis (MS) patients, one and two months after diagnosis. The Symptom Distress Scale, which includes a measure of fatigue on a five point scale (1—could not feel more tired; 5—not at all tired), was used to describe and compare symptoms. Both groups reported fatigue as distressing and identified it at both times as the most distressing symptom.

Krupp et al. (1988) compared fatigue in patients with MS to fatigue in a control group of healthy adults. Fatigue severity was measured by a visual analogue scale (VAS) and depression was measured by the Center for Epidemiologic Studies Depression Scale. From a series of open-ended interviews, they found that patients with MS were more likely to report that fatigue (a) prevented sustained physical activity, (b) worsened with heat, (c) interfered with physical function, (d) came on easily, (e) interfered with meeting responsibilities, and (f) caused frequent problems. Fatigue and depression were more common in the MS patients, but there was only a weak relationship between fatigue and depression in the group as a whole, and no relationship when both groups were analyzed separately. The investigators concluded that although there were similar features of fatigue in the MS and healthy group, fatigue in the MS group was more severe and more disabling than in the healthy group.

A group of 1,000 nurses were surveyed by Voith, Frank, and Pegg (1989) to define the characteristics of fatigue for the purpose of adopting fatigue as a nursing diagnosis. Although the survey had a low return rate (17.3 percent), the sample agreed on the following characteristics of the fatigued individual: (a) verbalizes fatigue, (b) is unable to maintain usual activity level, (c) has poor task performance, (d) has an impaired ability to concentrate, (e) feels irritable, and (f) expresses increased physical complaints.

Rhodes, Watson, and Hanson (1988) explored the relationship of selected symptoms to self-care abilities in patients receiving antineoplastic chemotherapy. Fatigue and weakness were found to be the most distressing symptoms causing the greatest amount of interference with self-care. In this research, the investigators agreed against fatigue as a nursing diagnosis because it was considered a subjective experience based on patients' perceptions rather than nurse identification. Pain, however, also a subjective experience, has been supported as a nursing diagnosis (McLane, 1987). More information about fatigue must be gathered before a final judgment can be made.

Piper (1988) indicated that the best way to measure fatigue is to ask people to describe how they feel and what they experience. She found that patients often fail to mention fatigue unless they are asked. Because family members are more likely to notice changes in behavioral patterns that might suggest fatigue, Piper suggested that families be included in the patient assessment process.

Clinical research is beginning to provide practitioners with data about the fatigue experience. Most research suggests that fatigue is distressing and interferes with functional ability. It is not known whether tiredness is a universal experience or whether there are cultural differences in the way people deal with fatigue. In order to understand the characteristics and patterns of fatigue, specific patient populations who are known to experience fatigue must be studied. This particular study focused on patients with congestive heart failure related to myocardial injury.

CONCEPTUAL FRAMEWORK

According to Levine (1973), fatigue is a manifestation of the body's attempt to heal itself. Fatigue occurs when the energy supply is unable to meet the energy demand. In illness, fatigue results from the body using its energy for healing (Levine, 1989). Fatigue exacts a toll on the emotional and physical well-being of the patient, particularly those with congestive heart failure.

Levine's Conservation Model (1973) was used as a basis for the development of this study. This model was chosen because of its focus on wholeness and the use of the scientific process at the bedside to assess the need for nursing care. According to Levine's model, individuals respond to internal and external environmental stimuli in an integrated yet singular fashion. When individuals are unable to adapt to the stimuli, they seek nursing care. The nurse's goal is to promote adaptation and to maintain the "wholeness" of the patient. The conservation principles are used by the nurse to identify interventions that will help the patients restore their perceptions of themselves as integrated or whole. In this study, the four conservation principles (energy conservation, structural integrity, personal integrity, and social integrity) served as the framework for the identification of study variables. It was expected that this approach would help maintain the patients' integrity.

The sensation of fatigue is a perception of a complex interplay of somatic and psychologic factors (Piper, 1986). With Levine's four conservation principles as a guideline, the nurse is able to anticipate many manifestations of the patient's fatigue experience:

(a) rapid heart rate, elevated temperature, low hemoglobin, and elevated blood sugar (energy conservation); (b) physical injury (structural integrity); (c) reduced self-worth (personal integrity); and (d) inability to socialize at the pre-illness level (social integrity).

PURPOSE

The objectives of this study were:

1. to describe the fatigue experience in patients with congestive heart failure related to myocardial injury;
2. to determine the relationship between selected objective parameters and the severity of fatigue in the patient with congestive heart failure related to myocardial injury;
3. to determine whether the fatigue experience described by patients with congestive heart failure related to myocardial injury has the same characteristics as the nursing diagnosis of fatigue described by NANDA; and
4. to demonstrate to staff nurses how existing procedures (assessment) and routinely collected data (vital signs, electrolytes, hemoglobin) can be used for research.

This paper addresses the first, second, and fourth objectives.

METHODS

A descriptive approach was used to assess and describe the fatigue experience of a sample of 23 patients who met the criteria for admission into the study. Admission criteria included (a) a diagnosis of congestive heart failure related to myocardial injury, (b) a sufficient level of alertness and orientation according to the patient record and the staff nurse's assessment, and (c) an ability to speak and understand English. Patients were excluded if they had congestive heart failure related to circulatory failure, if their primary nurse felt the patient was not a good interview candidate, or if the patient was in an intensive care unit.

Instruments

The Fatigue Interview Schedule (FIS) was developed by the investigator (this author) to assess the patients' perceptions of fatigue. The dimensions of fatigue identified by Piper (1988) were used as a basis for the development of open-ended questions (table 17-1). The FIS was examined by two clinical specialists and five graduate students who judged the effectiveness of the questions to elicit information about the seven dimensions of fatigue. The five graduate students, who were familiar with Levine's Conservation Model, were also asked to determine whether the questions were consistent with nursing's goal to promote wholeness according to the four conservation principles. They agreed that the questions would accomplish this task.

The Congestive Heart Failure Data Tool (CHFDT) was developed by the investigator to collect the data recorded on the patients' charts that has been suggested (Levine, 1973) to represent energy balance. The tool included variables that were routinely collected for all CHF patients admitted to an acute care hospital: vital signs, hemoglobin, blood gases, and blood glucose. If ejection fraction (EF) was known from previous admissions, it was recorded as a measure of structural integrity (table 17-2).

Table 17-1
Fatigue Dimensions and Interview Questions

Piper Dimensions[a]	Schaefer Questions
Temporal	When do you get fatigued? How long does this feeling of fatigue last?
Severity	Severity of fatigue on the Visual Analogue Scale?
Emotional	How do you feel about being fatigued?
Sensory	How do you feel about being fatigued? Does anything else happen to you when you are fatigued?
Evaluative	What does fatigue mean to you? What do you think causes the fatigue?
Associated symptoms	Does anything else happen to you when you are fatigued?
Relief	What do you do to relieve the fatigue?

[a] Piper, B. (1988). Fatigue self report scale developed. *Reflections, 14*(2), 11.

Table 17-2
Study Variables According to Levine's
Conservation Principles

Principle	Variable
Energy Conservation	Heart Rate
	Temperature
	Hemoglobin
	Blood Gases
	Blood Glucose
Structural Integrity	Ejection Fraction
Personal Integrity	Self-worth (How the patients feel about being fatigued)
Social Integrity	Ability to socialize (How the patients feel about being fatigued and whether anything else happens to them when they are fatigued)

Procedures

Potential subjects were identified through a review of the kardexes on the unit where the majority of patients with CHF were admitted. The primary nurses were asked to validate the diagnosis and to assess each patient's ability to take part in the interview. The purpose and nature of the study was explained to the patients. After the patients' questions were satisfactorily answered, written informed consent was obtained. Before the interview began, the investigator asked the patients to give their own definitions of fatigue. The Institutional Review Board recommended that this question be included to assure that the patients and the researcher were talking about the same phenomenon. After completing the interview, the investigator recorded the objective data on the CHFDT. The primary nurses were notified when the interviews were completed, and any care-related issues were referred to them.

Qualitative data were analyzed using content analysis of words representing descriptors of the fatigue experience. The Stat-Packets microcomputer program (Walonick, 1987) was used to analyze all quantitative data.

RESULTS

Thirty-four patients met the criteria for admission into the study from June 1989 to February 1990. Eight patients were excluded for a variety of reasons. One patient could not see the VAS, three were off the floor when the researcher was available, one patient was having a bad day, two patients had other illnesses that were confounding variables, and one patient whose EF was 15 percent fell asleep during the interview. Three patients refused to participate because of bad experiences they had had in the past after signing consent forms for diagnostic procedures. The remaining 23 patients, 12 men and 11 women, agreed to participate. Their ages ranged from 53 to 85 with a mean age of 69 (standard deviation [SD] = 8.2). At the time of the interview, patients had been hospitalized for an average of eight days (SD = 5.47; range = 1–21). The means, standard deviations, and ranges of all study variables can be found in table 17-3. Thirteen patients were fatigued

Table 17-3
Means, Standard Deviations, and Ranges of Study Variables

Variable	Mean	Standard Deviation	Range
Length of stay	8.13	5.47	1–21
Pulse rate	85	16.64	60–125
Number of medications	10	2.6	6–16
Temperature	97.7	1.3	96–100
Oxygen saturation	93.11	6.7	70–99
pH	7.42	.09	7.12–7.54
PCO2	37.11	10.57	20–62
PO2	74.47	19.9	51–121
HCO3	24.29	5.88	15–38
Hemoglobin	12.6	1.58	10–16
Hematocrit	38.82	4.55	31.4–48.6
Ejection Fraction	12	7.3	10–20
Age	69	8.2	53–85
Systolic Blood Pressure	131.75	28.6	80–185
Diastolic Blood Pressure	74.43	11.7	55–105
Respirations	22	4.96	12–32
Glucose	196.17	138.2	93–172
Number of illnesses	6.08	2.29	2–10
Severity of fatigue[a]	71.21	22.38	27–100

[a] Measured using the Fatigue Visual Analogue Scale. Low fatigue 1–33, Moderate fatigue 34–66, High fatigue 67–100.

on admission to the hospital, and 17 patients said that their fatigue occurred only once in a while. The remaining six stated that they were tired all the time.

To examine the variables relative to their influence on perceived severity of fatigue, a correlation matrix was created. Of the three variables that had a significant relationship to severity of fatigue, ejection fraction was the only variable with a strong significant relationship (table 17-4). Although a regression analysis of the independent variables on the dependent variable of fatigue might provide an indication of the predictors of fatigue, the large number of variables and the small sample in this study would make any significant predictor impossible to identify.

Analysis of the qualitative data indicated that 18 of the 23 participants defined fatigue as being tired. Other definitions included "being weak through and through," lack of energy, not being able to move around, and being "played out." Reasons for fatigue fell into two categories: stress and physical activity (table 17-5). Patient-initiated treatment for fatigue consisted primarily of rest or sleep and diversional activities (table 17-6). When asked

Table 17-4
Correlation of Independent Variables
With Severity of Fatigue

Variable	r	p	df
Ejection fraction	−.72	< .05	5
pH	−.42	< .05	22
Oxygen saturation	−.43	< .05	22
Age	−.14	NS	22
Hemoglobin	.14	NS	22
Hematocrit	.18	NS	22
PCO2	−.19	NS	22
Systolic Blood Pressure	−.18	NS	16
Diastolic Blood Pressure	.14	NS	22
Respirations	−.06	NS	16
PO2	−.09	NS	22
Number of medications	.30	NS	22
Pulse	.10	NS	16
Number of illnesses	.27	NS	22
Glucose	.20	NS	22
HCO3	−.24	NS	22

Note: NS = Not significant; r = correlation; p = probability; df = degrees of freedom.

Table 17-5
When Patients Get Fatigued

Category	Reasons for Fatigue
Stress	Stress in life
	Being "hyper"
Physical activity	Cleaning
	Walking up steps
	Washing myself
	Going to the bathroom
	Walking around
	Playing golf
	Exerting myself
	Dressing

what they thought caused their fatigue, nine of the 23 patients said it was their heart condition and seven patients said they had no idea why they were so tired. When asked how they felt about being fatigued, several indicated that they just took it in stride. One individual explained simply that she was not as young as she used to be. Ten of the 23 subjects stated that being fatigued was an annoyance, a frustration, a bitter disappointment, scary, and made them angry. Other symptoms associated with fatigue included nausea, loss of appetite, shortness of breath, light headedness, and feeling "blah."

Table 17-6
Patient-Initiated Supportive Interventions for Fatigue

Category	Behavior
Sleep and/or rest	Go to bed/lie down
	Nap
	Take it easy
	Sit and relax
	Sleep
Diversion	Think about pleasant things
	Do crossword puzzles
	Listen to music
	Read

On the average, the subjects were taking 10 prescribed medications (SD = 2.6), including as-needed drugs, and had six diagnoses (SD = 2.29) in addition to the congestive heart failure related to myocardial damage. All patients rated the severity of their fatigue on the VAS. A mean score of 71.21 fell within the upper quartile with a variance (SD = 22.38) that suggests group heterogeneity. Fifty-seven percent rated the fatigue as high, 35 percent as medium, and 8 percent as low.

THE FATIGUE EXPERIENCE

Because the focus of this study was to describe the fatigue experience, the data should contribute to the development of theory through the description and increased understanding of the phenomenon of fatigue. A collective description of fatigue was expressed best by one patient:

> Fatigue means my whole being is tired. This tiredness penetrates the whole bone structure; you feel it in the very marrow of your bones. It is total physical tiredness, and on top of that is mental tiredness. It's like an undercurrent that undermines your thinking. Your body is wearing out. The weight of fatigue is in the shadows. If I rest, the fatigue will overwhelm me.

Most patients did not have the ability to express themselves as poetically, but they did perceive themselves as being tired. Tiredness was a singular feeling, expressed as a feeling involving the whole being; this reinforced the notion that these patients do see themselves as whole.

All patients in this study identified interventions that helped reduce the feeling of fatigue. These interventions were similar to the patient-initiated fatigue interventions identified by patients with cancer (Piper et al., 1989) (table 17-7). However, patients in this study did not identify exercise or nutritional approaches to their fatigue. This may have been due in part to the group's higher mean age. For example, exercise may not have been perceived as possible because of bone related changes or simply because of age.

Table 17-7
Patient-Initiated Interventions

Cancer Patients[a]	CHF Patients
Rest	Go to bed/lie down
Nap	Nap
Alter activities	Take it easy
Sit and/or lie down	Sit and relax
Read	Read
Walk and/or exercise	
Distraction	Think about pleasant things
	Do crossword puzzles
	Listen to music
Relax	Sit and relax
Sleep	Sleep
Improve Nutrition	
Alter Environment	
Socialize	
Symptoms	

[a]These interventions are from Piper, B.F., et al. (1989). Recent advances in the management of biotherapy-related side effects: Fatigue. *Oncology Nursing Forum*, 16(6) (Supplement), 27–34.

Additionally, the open-ended questions did not lead the patients to focus on this information.

In this study the majority of patients were fatigued on admission to the hospital, and rated fatigue as high. However, none of the patients had sought medical attention because of their fatigue. Although reasons for seeking health care were not the focus of this study, whether or not the fatigue was documented on admission was assessed, and it was found not to have been an admission criterion. One can assume that unless the nurse asks about fatigue, the patient does not see it as a problem and will not voluntarily offer the information. Furthermore, these patients may have perceived fatigue as a result of getting old, and many may have accepted the condition as normal. The high mean score of fatigue severity may be reflective of the tendency for subjects to cluster responses in the upper quartile of the VAS and, therefore, may not represent a true value. Fatigue as the result of anemia associated with chronic illness is not supported by the results of this study. The mean hemoglobin of 12.6 (SD = 1.58) was well within normal limits.

A Description of Fatigue

CONCEPTUAL MODEL CONSIDERATIONS

The four conservation principles of Levine's Conservation Model are energy conservation, structural integrity, personal integrity, and social integrity. These principles were used to identify the characteristics of fatigue and recommend therapeutic nursing interventions (table 17–8).

Energy conservation involves the balancing of energy supply and demand to avoid excessive fatigue. The nurse's goal is to oversee the proper disbursement of energy, allowing for activity in the range of individual capability. Patients in this study were tired, devoid of the energy to do some of the things they were used to doing. Their energy output was reduced, both physically and emotionally. While this was discouraging to them, rest and enjoyable diversional activities helped them through the fatigue. They modified the internal and external environment to provide themselves with some relief, although each person did not necessarily include both rest and diversional activities in their

Table 17-8
The Structure of Fatigue: Use of
Levine's Conservation Principles

Problem	Intervention
Energy Conservation	
Tired	Rest
	Distraction therapy
Structural Integrity	
Reduced ejection fraction	Rest
	Monitor response to drugs
Personal Integrity	
Frustrated	Teach
	Acknowledge problems
	Support through changes
Social Integrity	
Reduced ability to engage in activities	Plan
	Rest

self-identified prescriptions. Nurses can suggest the use of distraction techniques within the abilities of the patient while assessing for an organismic response that represents energy balance (such as normal heart rate).

Most of the physiological measures of the patients in this study were normal, although they tended to be on the low normal side. It is possible that a larger sample would have produced significant relationships between fatigue severity and other study variables such as temperature and number of medications. Normally the heart rate is a fairly good measure of energy use; in this study the mean heart rate was normal. This normal response may represent the stage of adaptive resistance described by Selye (1976). In this stage, an enlargement and multiplication of preexisting cell elements without qualitative change occurs (Selye, 1976). At the same time tissue readjustment or transformation redevelop in order to allow the patient to perform diverse functions (Leidy, 1989). Organismically, normal vital signs result.

The conservation of *structural integrity* involves maintaining or restoring the structure of the body in order to prevent physical breakdown and to promote healing. Although the physiological measures in this group were normal, a strong significant relationship was found between ejection fraction and severity of fatigue. Caution is exercised in the interpretation of this relationship because of the small sample size; however, the correlation was significant. There may be a level of ejection fraction that falls outside each individual's unique adaptive abilities that is representative of exhaustion, the final stage of Selye's (1976) stress response. Clinically this may explain why the patient with an ejection fraction of 15 percent fell asleep during the interview.

Nurses cannot alter the effect of a low ejection fraction, but they can provide supportive therapy to maintain the status quo. Careful patterning of activity and rest and the monitoring of medication for unwanted side effects may help reduce stress on the myocardium.

The conservation of *personal integrity* involves the maintenance or restoration of the patient's sense of identity and self-worth. Eight patients in this study had no idea why they were feeling so tired and were frustrated by their inability to do what they were used to doing. Helping patients understand the reasons for feeling so tired might enable them to deal realistically with their imposed life-style changes. Nurses can help patients acknowledge their problems; they can explain the fatigue response (heart fails to pump adequately, reducing the amount of blood and nutrients that are delivered to the tissues), and they can help patients plan activities that enable them to maintain some control over their lives.

The conservation of *social integrity* means acknowledging the patient as a social being. Levine (1973) tells us that patients' lives take on meaning in the context of their environments. Planned outings or other social activities may be successful as diversional therapy for some patients and may reduce or change their perceptions of fatigue. One patient in this study stated that she could never plan to go out with her friends because she never knew if she would have the energy to do so. The nurse can help patients plan their activities with scheduled rest beforehand. However, there are some whose tiredness may never go away. More dramatic measures may be required for these individuals to maintain their sense of wholeness.

METHODOLOGICAL CONSIDERATIONS

Acute fatigue is generally defined as normal or expected fatigue of short duration. It appears intermittently and serves a protective function (Piper et al., 1989). Chronic fatigue is considered excessive and constant, and it may be cumulative and may last for more than a month (Piper et al., 1989). Some investigators consider fatigue chronic if it lasts more than a few days (Manu, Matthews, & Lane, 1988). In this study, acute fatigue was defined as fatigue occurring once in a while; fatigue was considered chronic if it lasted all the time. These simplistic definitions may misrepresent the true nature of fatigue variations.

The majority of patients in this study said that their fatigue occurred only once in a while. This assessment of fatigue was based primarily on patient recall and may have been somewhat distorted. Piper et al. (1989) have noted that research still needs to determine whether chronic and acute fatigue are different syndromes or whether they are simply variations of the same problem. Until this is determined, what the patient tells us must be considered reliable and valid (Leininger, 1984). As Levine (1973) has indicated, fatigue is a cue that the body is experiencing an energy imbalance, regardless of its nature, and the nurse's goal is to help the patient adapt by creating a balance of energy supply and demand.

Although the VAS is an appealing instrument for the measure of subjective feelings, it is not without methodological problems. For most individuals, the concept of a line representing feelings is not difficult to understand. However, the older population, such as the sample in this study, has been reported to have difficulty with the tool (Gift, 1989). Two individuals in this study did not understand what was meant by marking the line at the point that represented the severity of their fatigue. Their confusion was alleviated when the investigator used the numbers one to ten to explain the various possible points on the scale. Therefore, in this study the measure of the VAS may be a measure of discrete points rather than a continuum and the data ordinal rather than interval. Dividing the responses into quartiles accounts for some of the error introduced by treating ordinal data as interval data. In this study most of the patients rated their fatigue in the upper quartile, which represented severe fatigue (Lee & Kieckhefer, 1989). An additional limitation of the VAS is that it has been found to be most reliable as a measure of change, and in this study it was used to study the single measure of fatigue.

The tools developed by the investigator for this study have limited reliability and validity, which confines the generalizability of the findings. However, content validity for a descriptive study may be sufficient, since generalizability was not the purpose of this level of study.

The patients had a mean age of 69 (SD = 8.2). Older patients frequently require special attention as participants in research because of normal changes that occur with age such as failure in hearing or sight (Gueldner & Hanner, 1989). Anticipating such problems, the researcher read the consent forms to the patients unless they requested otherwise, and she used open-ended questions in an interview setting rather than questionnaires requiring completion by the subjects. In order to avoid the question of literacy, the researcher read the questions out loud, positioning the paper so the subject could read along with her. Although older patients frequently have difficulty with recent recall, none of the patients in this study had any difficulty remembering how tired they were.

IMPLICATIONS

From the perspective of the Conservation Model, fatigue is a symptom of impending or existing problems that result from an imbalance of energy supply and demand. Fatigue can be interpreted as beneficial or protective. It is a warning for the individual to do something about the cause of fatigue—to rest, eat more nutritious meals, or exercise regularly. Fatigue that persists and requires medical attention also serves a protective function because it causes the individual to seek health care (Piper et al., 1989). In either case, the nurse continues to focus care on the maintenance of wholeness and facilitation of adaptation by helping to bring the patient's energy supply and demand back into balance.

The sample in this study did not initiate the identification of fatigue or discuss it as problematic with their primary nurses; they talked about it in response to the researcher's questions. Patients indicated that they really did not expect to be able to do as much as they could in the past, simply because they were older. The notion that fatigue is relative and acceptable to this population requires further study.

Levine (1973) notes that individuals are past-aware and future-oriented. Past life-styles influence an individual's perceptions of phenomena in the present. This holds true for fatigue as well. Individuals who were not active in the past may be less aware of fatigue. The patients in this study had multiple illnesses and were taking an average of six medications. Both the illnesses and the medications could have influenced their perceptions of fatigue.

The findings in this study suggest that fatigue may be an unspoken problem for the elderly. Although patients did not offer information about their fatigue until asked, a physician present during one of the interviews indicated that fatigue was the major problem of all the CHF patients he saw in his office (Dr. Glen Short, personal communication, August 27, 1989). This insight suggests that questions about fatigue and what helps to alleviate it should be part of the initial interaction between nurses and their patients and patient family members.

Some patients may never be completely relieved of their fatigue. A number of subjects in this study did not understand the cause of their own tiredness. Nursing interventions may be as simple as helping individuals to understand the cause of their fatigue and helping them maintain a balanced life-style in order to reduce the effects of their tiredness.

There is still more to learn about fatigue in this population and others. In-depth interviews may clarify the multiple manifestations and meanings of fatigue and the differences between types of patients. For example, it is very unlikely that fatigue in an ill child is like that experienced by the subjects in this study. Children have had very little time to be past-aware.

Surveys that include questions related to dietary habits and exercise may help expand the understanding of the nature of fatigue. Given the subjective nature *and* the relativity of the experience, it is doubtful that fatigue will hold up under rigorous testing as a diagnosis. It is an experience to which nurses help patients adapt, and the effects of their interventions for this group in particular (rest and/or exercise, nutrition, distraction, and socialization) require further analysis.

SUMMARY

Congestive heart failure is associated with overwhelming tiredness, which interferes with functional ability. The severity of fatigue in this patient population is subjective and may be relative to age and past activity level. Levine's Conservation Model is useful for the study of fatigue in the practice setting. The conservation principles should be used in the design of therapeutic measures because the goal of these principles is to maintain the patient's integrity.

REFERENCES

Aistars, J. (1987). Fatigue in the cancer patient: A conceptual approach to a clinical problem. *Oncology Nursing Forum, 14*(6), 25-30.

Bruera, E., & MacDonald, R. N. (1988). Overwhelming fatigue in advanced cancer. *American Journal of Nursing, 88*(1), 99-100.

Carroll-Johnson, R. M. (Ed.). (1989). *Classification of nursing diagnosis: Proceedings of the eighth conference.* Philadelphia: J.B. Lippincott.

Fields, W. L., & Loveridge, C. (1988). Critical thinking and fatigue: How do nurses on 8 & 12 hour shifts compare? *Nursing Economics, 6*(4), 189-191.

Gift, A. (1989). Visual analogue scales: Measures of subjective phenomenon. *Nursing Research, 38*(5), 286-287.

Gregersen, R. A. (1988). Fatigue in the cardiac surgical patient. *Progress in Cardiovascular Nursing, 3*(4), 106-111.

Gueldner, S., & Hanner, M. B. (1989). Methodological issues related to gerontological nursing research. *Nursing Research, 38*(3), 183-185.

Haylock, P. J., & Hart, L. K. (1979). Fatigue in patients receiving localized radiation. *Cancer Nursing, 2,* 461-467.

Kellum, M. D. (1986). Fatigue. In M. M. Jacobs & W. Geels (Eds.). *Signs and symptoms in nursing: Intervention and management* (pp. 103-118). Philadelphia: J.B. Lippincott.

Krupp, L. B., Alvarez, L. A., LaRocca, N. G., & Scheinberg, L. C. (1988). Fatigue in multiple sclerosis. *Archives of Neurology, 45,* 435-437.

Lee, K. A., & Kieckhefer, G. M. (1989). Measuring human responses using visual analogue scales. *Western Journal of Nursing Research, 11*(1), 128-132.

Leidy, M. K. (1989). A physiological analysis of stress and chronic illness. *Journal of Advanced Nursing, 14,* 868-876.

Leininger, M. M. (1984). *Care: The essence of nursing and health.* Thorofare, NJ: Slack.

Levine, M. E. (1973). *Introduction to clinical nursing* (2nd ed.). Philadelphia: F.A. Davis.

Levine, M. E. (1989). The conservation principles of nursing twenty years later. In J. P. Reihl-Sisca (Ed.). *Conceptual models for nursing practice* (3rd ed.) (pp. 325–348). Norwalk, CT: Appleton & Lange.

Manu, P., Matthews, D. A., & Lane, T. J. (1988). The frequency of the chronic fatigue syndrome in patients with symptoms of persistent fatigue. *Annals of Internal Medicine, 148,* 554–556.

McCorkle, R. (1981, August). Social support and symptom distress in two samples with life-threatening diseases. Paper presented at the American Cancer Society Second Conference on Cancer Nursing Research, Seattle, WA.

McLane, A. M. (1987). *Classification of nursing diagnosis: Proceedings of the seventh conference.* St. Louis: C.V. Mosby.

Piper, B. (1986). Fatigue. In V. K. Carrieri & A. M. Lindsey (Eds.). *Pathophysiological phenomena in nursing: Human response to illness* (pp. 219–234). Philadelphia: W.B. Saunders.

Piper, B. (1988). Fatigue self report scale developed. *Reflections, 14*(2), 11.

Piper, B. F., Lindsey, A. M., & Dodd, M. J. (1987). Fatigue mechanisms in cancer patients: Developing nursing theory. *Oncology Nursing Forum, 14*(6), 17–23.

Piper, B. F., Rieger, P. T., Brophy, L., Haeuber, D., Hood, L. E., Lyver, A., & Sharp, E. (1989). Recent advances in the management of biotherapy-related side effects: Fatigue. *Oncology Nursing Forum, 16*(6) (Supplement), 27–34.

Potempa, K., Lopex, M., Reid, C., & Lawson, L. (1986). Chronic fatigue. *Image: Journal of International Nursing Scholarship, 18*(4), 165–169.

Reich, S. G. (1986). The tired patient: Psychological versus organic causes. *Hospital Medicine, 22*(7), 142–154.

Rhodes, V. A., Watson, P. M., & Hanson, B. (1988). Patients' descriptions of the influence of tiredness and weakness on self-care abilities. *Cancer Nursing, 11*(3), 186–194.

Selye, H. (1976). *The stress of life.* New York: McGraw-Hill.

Srivastava, R. H. (1986). Fatigue in the renal patient. *American Neurological Nurses Association Journal, 13*(5), 246–249.

Voith, A. M., Frank, A. M., & Pegg, J. S. (1989). Validation of fatigue as a nursing diagnosis. In R. M. Carroll-Johnson (Ed.). *Classification of nursing diagnosis: Proceedings of the eighth conference* (pp. 453–458). Philadelphia: J.B. Lippincott.

Walonick, D. S. (1987). Stat-Packets statistical analysis packets for Lotus worksheets (Version 1.0). Minneapolis, MN: Walonick Associates.

Part 8

The Neuman Systems Model

18

The Neuman Systems Model: A Theory for Practice

Betty M. Neuman

As evidenced by the literature, an increasingly comprehensive view of client care is coming into being. The major influence of this change in view is the maturing of the nursing profession, with increased concern for issues of image, autonomy, and accountability. Information overload alone reflects the need for a comprehensive system within which to organize and structure nursing phenomena. The Neuman Systems Model is increasingly being recognized as fulfilling these needs as it has a universal quality and appeal, which adapts well to all cultures.

This chapter will present the components of the Neuman Systems Model and tools for the model's implementation abstracted from the Neuman text (1989). The explanation will be related to the four accepted concepts of nursing—man (client), environment, health, and nursing—and will include materials presented at the spring 1990 conference in Florida. This chapter includes some recently developed views of the author (Neuman, 1990): (1) wellness as defined within the systems perspective, (2) a generic guide for use of the model in acute and critical care, and (3) a look to the future utility of the model for nursing.

MODELS AND NURSING

Models have long been used as a base for scientific thinking by other disciplines, providing a particular view from which to organize the phenomena of the field. Nursing models are proving their value as well and are thought of as symbolic representations of reality. Many nursing models relate to the four accepted concepts of nursing. During the past decade, theorists have expanded their nursing models to become congruent with these four general concepts that comprise the discipline of nursing.

THE NEUMAN SYSTEMS MODEL

The Neuman Systems Model was developed and used in 1970 at UCLA as a tool for graduate nursing students who requested a course that would introduce the variables from which they would later choose a specific area for clinical specialization. A two-year student evaluation initially reflected the value of this course and the Neuman Systems Model to students.

The Neuman Model presents a way of viewing clients holistically and multidimensionally within a systemic perspective. It considers all the variables affecting a client's possible or actual responses to environmental stressors. It illustrates the composite of five interacting variables—physiological, psychological, sociocultural, developmental, and spiritual—which ideally function harmoniously and stably in response to the internal and external environmental stressors influencing the client at a given point in time. The model is based on the concept of stress and on possible or actual reaction to stress. The entire structure of the client system, with identifiable parts, is maintained by the interrelationship of system components that evolve out of the dynamics of the open system.

The model is dynamic in that it is based on the client's continuous interaction with environmental stress factors occurring in both wellness and illness conditions. This model facilitates the uniqueness of the nursing profession in its consideration of all client system variables and its holistic, comprehensive approach to client situations. The dynamic nature of interactive, interdependent, and interrelated client system functioning requires multidimensional

Figure 18-1
The Neuman Systems Model

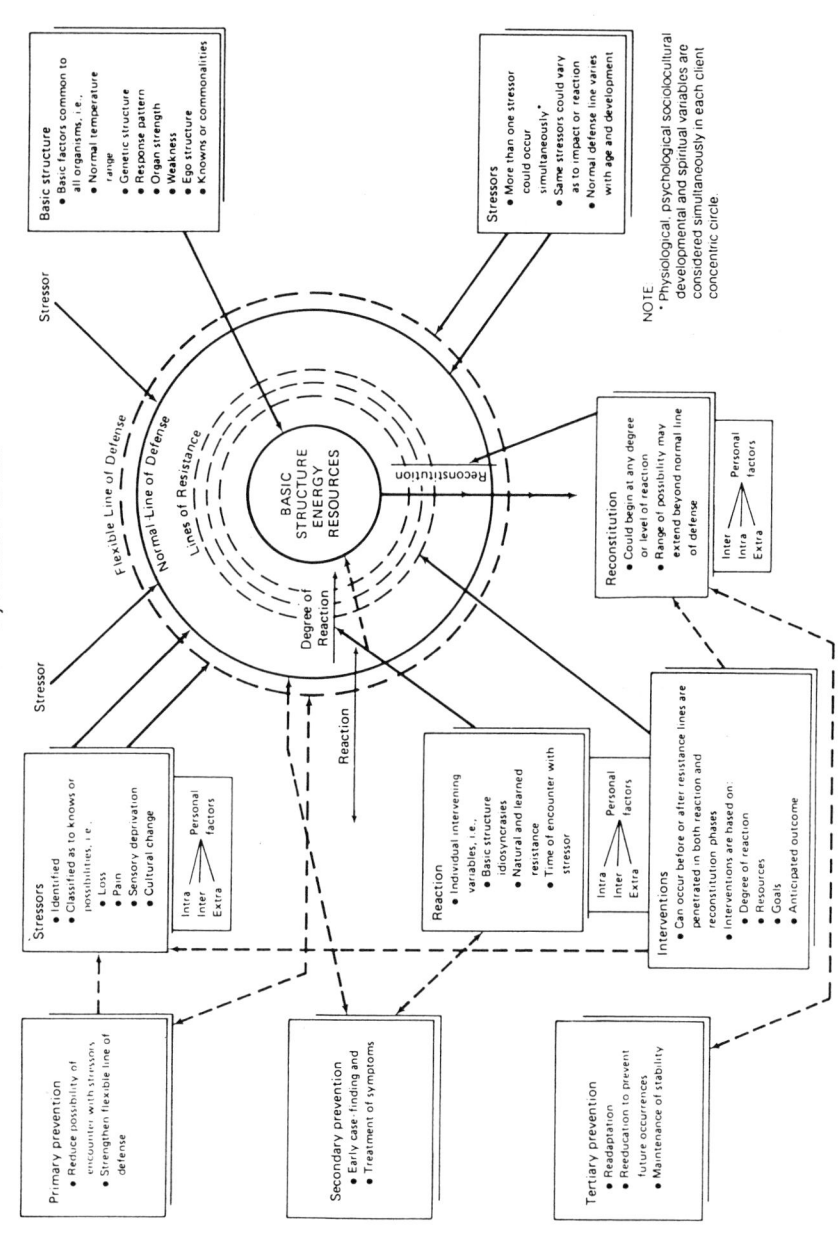

Copyright © 1970 by Betty Neuman. Reprinted by permission.

thinking and acting resulting in unique conceptions, roles, and creativity in organizing and using knowledge at all levels of nursing. The systems approach unifies nursing in terms of organization and structure of its parts relevant to both nursing and the larger health care system.

Figure 18-1, a diagram of the Neuman Systems Model, illustrates the model's correlation with the major concepts of nursing and provides direction for its use as an important organizing structure for the profession. The individual components of this diagram will be further explained in the following sections.

Client

The client/client system segment of the Neuman Systems Model (figure 18-2) shows the client as a dynamic system represented by concentric circles surrounding and protecting a basic structure.

Figure 18-2
Client/Client System

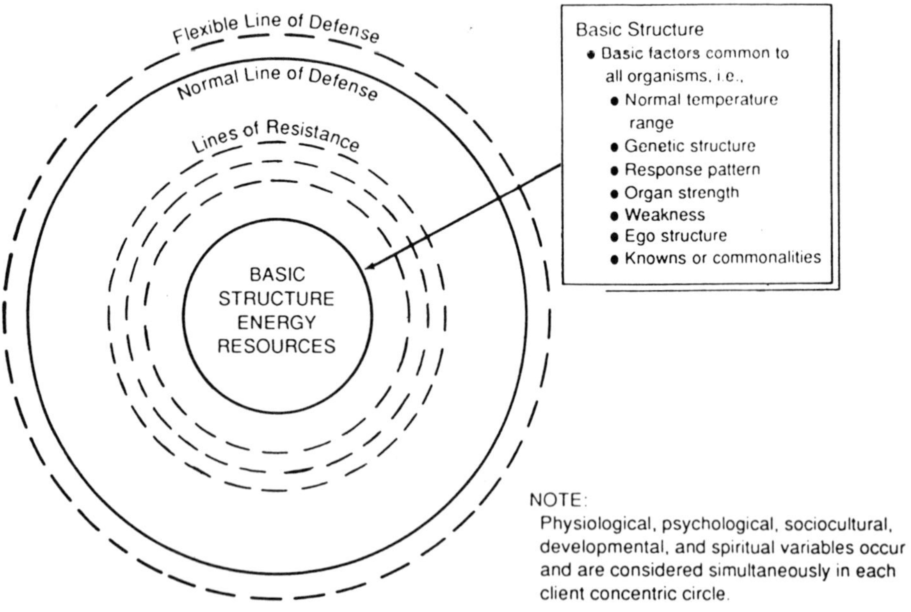

Flexible Line of Defense
Normal Line of Defense
Lines of Resistance
BASIC STRUCTURE ENERGY RESOURCES

Basic Structure
- Basic factors common to all organisms, i.e.,
  - Normal temperature range
  - Genetic structure
  - Response pattern
  - Organ strength
  - Weakness
  - Ego structure
  - Knowns or commonalities

NOTE:
Physiological, psychological, sociocultural, developmental, and spiritual variables occur and are considered simultaneously in each client concentric circle.

Reprinted from Neuman, B. (1989). *The Neuman Systems Model*. Norwalk, CT: Appleton & Lange. Reprinted by permission.

The outer system boundary, the flexible line of defense (broken circle) protects the normal line of defense (solid circle), which represents the usual wellness level. A reaction is caused by stressor invasion of the normal defense line. In a reaction, the lines of resistance are activated as resources for reversing illness symptoms. When these lines of resistance fail to reverse illness symptoms, stressor penetration of the basic structure may result in system energy depletion and death. All lines of defense and resistance have a protective function against environmental stressors occurring within a wide range of dynamic interactive elements, patterns, styles, and potentials of the five client system variables. The goal of the system is to maintain stability while constantly adjusting to the effects of internal and external stressors.

A system may be defined as an individual, family, group, community, or issue, as the same systemic principles apply. The system is the client.

Environment

Environment (figure 18-3) is broadly defined as all internal and external factors or influences surrounding the identified client system. These environmental influences are considered stressors; the outcome of their interaction with client system variables determines their nature as harmful or beneficial. Intrapersonal stressors are internal, that is, contained within the boundaries of the client system. Interpersonal and extrapersonal stressors are external and are either within immediate or more distal range of the client system. Environmental exchanges must be identified and evaluated as to their potential or actual outcome for the client system.

Health

Health or wellness is viewed as being on a continuum of wellness to illness (figure 18-4). In wellness, more energy is being stored than used and in illness, more energy is being used than is available. Energy flow is continuous between the client system and environment.

Health is equated with optimal client system stability, that is, the best possible health condition for any given time (figure 18-5).

Figure 18-3
Environment

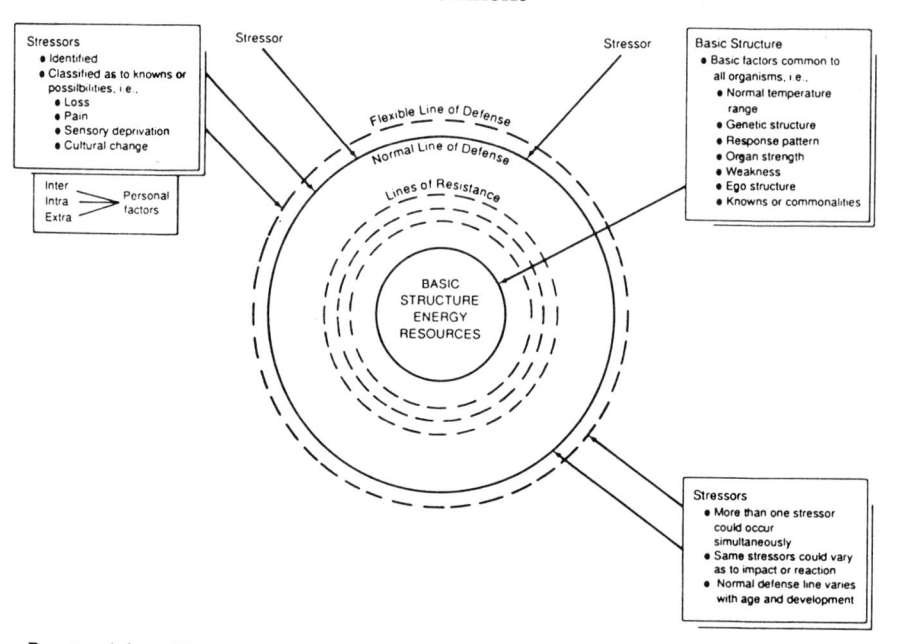

Stressors
- Identified
- Classified as to knowns or possibilities, i.e.,
  - Loss
  - Pain
  - Sensory deprivation
  - Cultural change

Inter / Intra / Extra → Personal factors

Stressor, Stressor

Flexible Line of Defense
Normal Line of Defense
Lines of Resistance

BASIC STRUCTURE ENERGY RESOURCES

Basic Structure
- Basic factors common to all organisms, i.e.,
  - Normal temperature range
  - Genetic structure
  - Response pattern
  - Organ strength
  - Weakness
  - Ego structure
  - Knowns or commonalities

Stressors
- More than one stressor could occur simultaneously
- Same stressors could vary as to impact or reaction
- Normal defense line varies with age and development

Reprinted from Neuman, B. (1989). *The Neuman Systems Model.* Norwalk, CT: Appleton & Lange. Reprinted by permission.

Figure 18-4
The Wellness-Illness Continuum

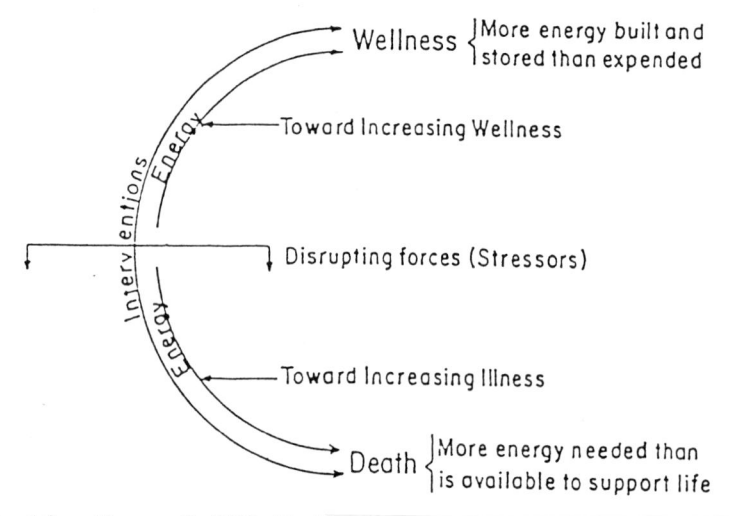

Wellness { More energy built and stored than expended

Toward Increasing Wellness

Interventions / Energy

Disrupting forces (Stressors)

Toward Increasing Illness

Death { More energy needed than is available to support life

Reprinted from Neuman, B. (1989). *The Neuman Systems Model.* Norwalk, CT: Appleton & Lange. Reprinted by permission.

Figure 18-5
Health

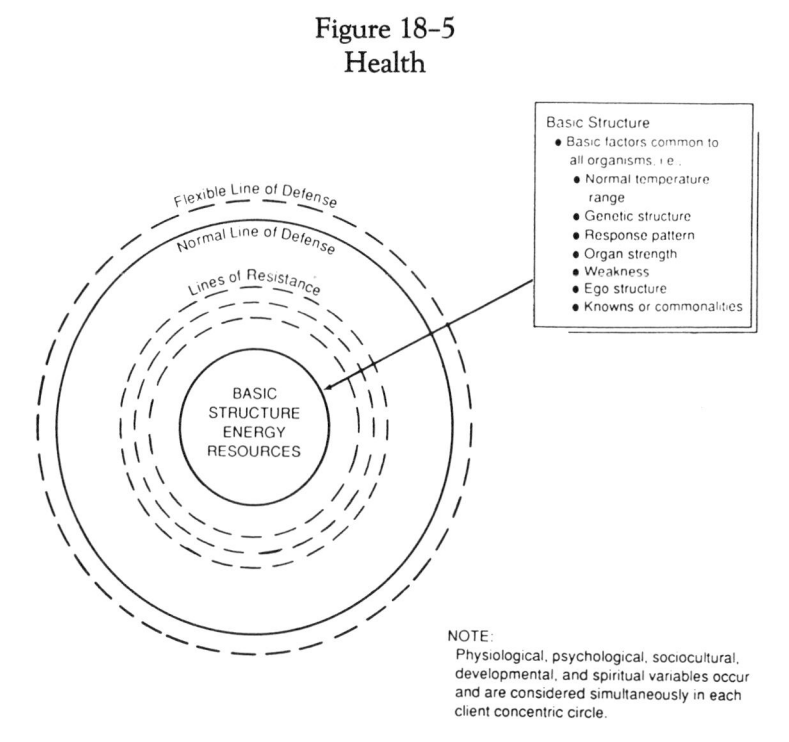

Basic Structure
- Basic factors common to all organisms, i.e.,
  - Normal temperature range
  - Genetic structure
  - Response pattern
  - Organ strength
  - Weakness
  - Ego structure
  - Knowns or commonalities

Flexible Line of Defense
Normal Line of Defense
Lines of Resistance
BASIC STRUCTURE ENERGY RESOURCES

NOTE: Physiological, psychological, sociocultural, developmental, and spiritual variables occur and are considered simultaneously in each client concentric circle.

Reprinted from Neuman, B. (1989). *The Neuman Systems Model*. Norwalk, CT: Appleton & Lange. Reprinted by permission.

Satisfactory and unsatisfactory adjustment to environmental stressors determines the wellness level. Health problems arise from unmet system needs related to the effects of stressors.

Nursing

The major concern for nursing is in keeping the client system stable through accuracy in assessment of effects and possible effects of environmental stressors and by assisting clients to make adjustments necessary for achievement of an optimal wellness level for a given point in time. Nursing actions are initiated to best retain, attain, and maintain optimal client health or wellness, using the three levels of prevention as interventions to keep the system stable (figure 18-6). Thus, the nurse creates a linkage between client, environment, health, and nursing.

Primary prevention (figure 18-7) is used to *retain* the client wellness state by protecting against stressor invasion of the normal line of defense which represents the usual (over time) health condition. As the flexible line of defense is strengthened, it resists both situational and on-going stressors, keeping the client system stable and thus free of illness symptoms. Primary prevention as intervention may also facilitate specific goals of health promotion and be used concomitant with secondary and/or tertiary preventive nursing actions.

Secondary prevention (figure 18-8) is used to *attain* wellness or treat illness symptoms. Secondary prevention as intervention protects the basic structure by strengthening the internal lines of resistance to reduce and/or reverse the reaction (illness symptoms) caused by stressor invasion of the normal line of

Figure 18-6
Nursing

Primary prevention
- Reduce possibility of encounter with stressors
- Strengthen flexible line of defense

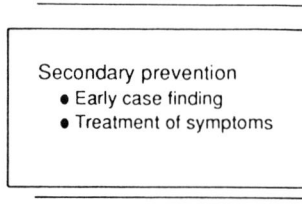

Secondary prevention
- Early case finding
- Treatment of symptoms

Tertiary prevention
- Readaptation
- Reeducation to prevent future occurrences
- Maintenance of stability

Inter
Intra → Personal factors
Extra

Interventions
- Can occur before or after resistance lines are penetrated in both reaction and reconstitution phases
- Interventions are based on:
  - Degree of reaction
  - Resources
  - Goals
  - Anticipated outcome

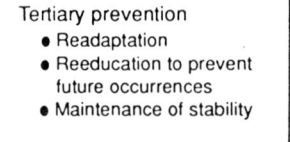

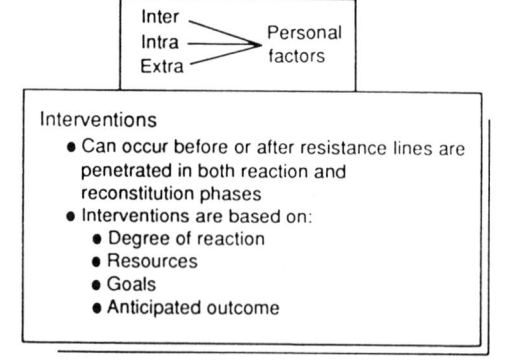

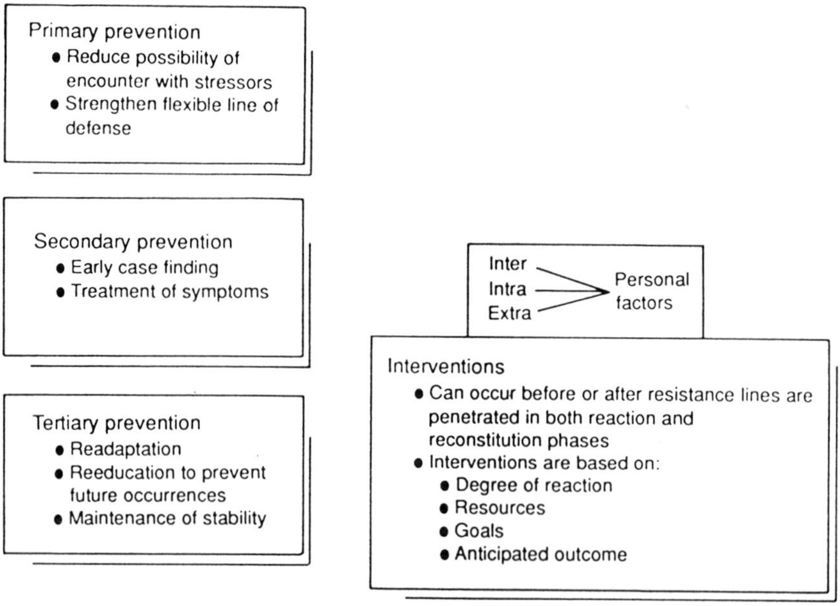

Reprinted from Neuman, B. (1989). *The Neuman Systems Model.* Norwalk, CT: Appleton & Lange. Reprinted by permission.

Figure 18-7
Format for Primary Prevention as Intervention Mode

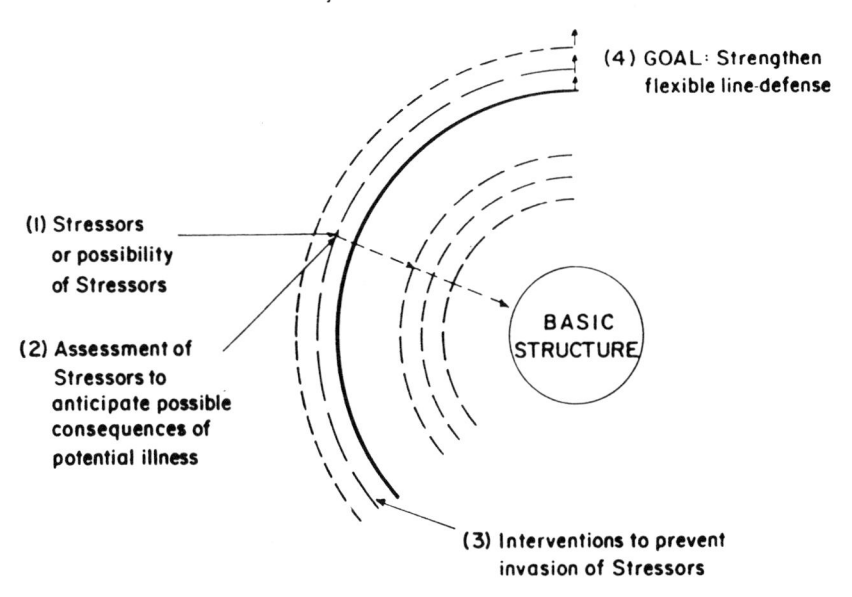

(1) Stressors or possibility of Stressors

(2) Assessment of Stressors to anticipate possible consequences of potential illness

(3) Interventions to prevent invasion of Stressors

(4) GOAL: Strengthen flexible line-defense

BASIC STRUCTURE

Copyright © 1980 by Betty Neuman. Reprinted by permission.

Figure 18-8
Format for Secondary Prevention as Intervention Mode

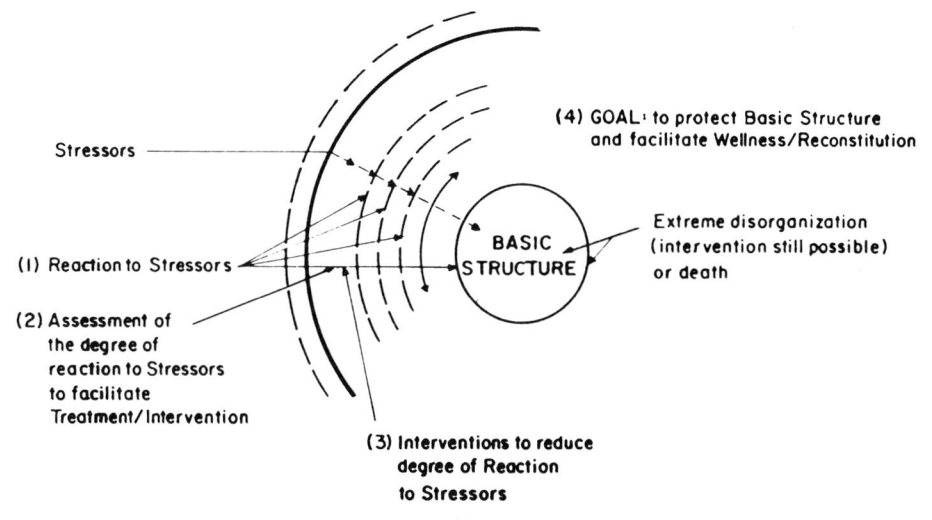

Stressors

(1) Reaction to Stressors

(2) Assessment of the degree of reaction to Stressors to facilitate Treatment/Intervention

(3) Interventions to reduce degree of Reaction to Stressors

(4) GOAL: to protect Basic Structure and facilitate Wellness/Reconstitution

BASIC STRUCTURE

Extreme disorganization (intervention still possible) or death

Copyright © 1980 by Betty Neuman. Reprinted by permission.

defense, or usual wellness level, reducing system stability. When secondary preventive actions fail, the basic structure is invaded, resulting in vital energy loss and possible death.

Tertiary prevention (figure 18-9) is used to *maintain* wellness following secondary preventive nursing actions. When reconstitution or client system stability becomes manifest, tertiary prevention as intervention may be begun to prevent regression and facilitate optimal client stability or wellness.

Use of all three preventions as interventions helps facilitate a dynamic state of client system adjustment to stressors (considering integration of all necessary factors) toward optimal use of existing resources for system stability or *wellness retention, attainment,* and *maintenance.* Table 18-1 illustrates nursing action in a format for prevention and intervention. Direction for nursing diagnosis, nursing goals, and nursing outcomes within the Neuman nursing process format are presented in table 18-2.

Figure 18-9
Format for Tertiary Prevention as Intervention Mode

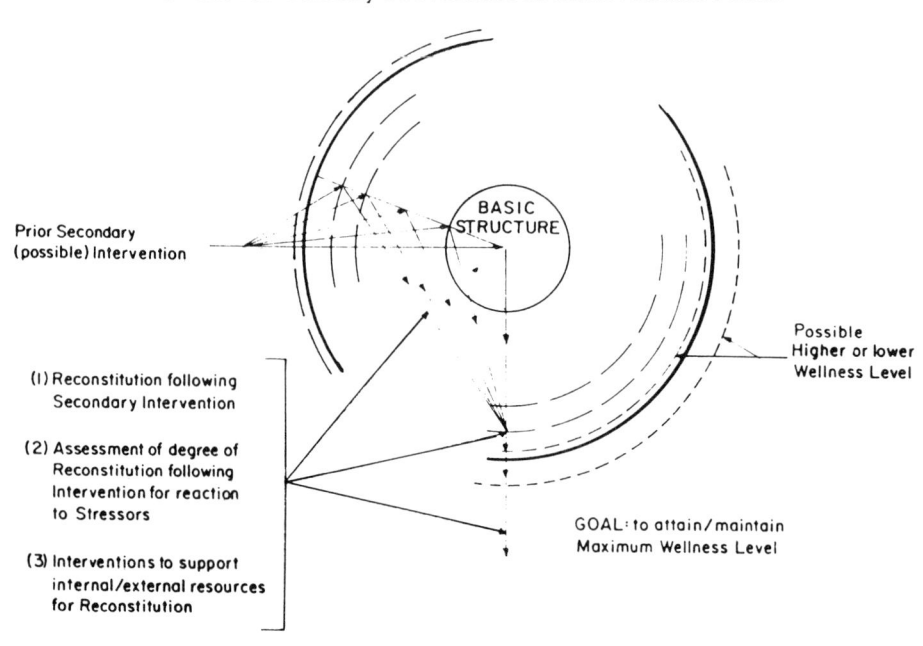

Prior Secondary (possible) Intervention

(1) Reconstitution following Secondary Intervention

(2) Assessment of degree of Reconstitution following Intervention for reaction to Stressors

(3) Interventions to support internal/external resources for Reconstitution

BASIC STRUCTURE

Possible Higher or lower Wellness Level

GOAL: to attain/maintain Maximum Wellness Level

Copyright © 1980 by Betty Neuman. Reprinted by permission.

Table 18-1
Format for Prevention as Intervention

Nursing Action		
Primary Prevention	**Secondary Prevention**	**Tertiary Prevention**
1. Classify stressors that threaten stability of the client/client system. Prevent stressor invasion.	1. Following stressor invasion, protect basic structure.	1. During reconstitution, attain and maintain maximum level of wellness or stability following treatment.
2. Provide information to retain or strengthen existing client/client system strengths.	2. Mobilize and optimize internal/external resources to attain stability and energy conservation.	2. Educate, reeducate, and/or reorient as needed.
3. Support positive coping and functioning.	3. Facilitate purposeful manipulation of stressors and reactions to stressors.	3. Support client/client system toward appropriate goals.
4. Desensitize existing or possible noxious stressors.	4. Motivate, educate, and involve client/client system in health care goals.	4. Coordinate and integrate health service resources.
5. Motivate toward wellness.	5. Facilitate appropriate treatment and intervention measures.	5. Provide primary and/or secondary preventive intervention as required.
6. Coordinate and integrate interdisciplinary theories and epidemiological input.	6. Support positive factors toward wellness.	
7. Educate or reeducate.	7. Promote advocacy by coordination and integration.	
8. Use stress as a positive intervention strategy.	8. Provide primary preventive intervention as required.	

Note: A first priority for nursing action in each of the areas of prevention as intervention is to determine the nature of stressors and their threat to the client/client system. Some general categorical functions for nursing action are initiation, planning, organization, monitoring, coordinating, implementing, integrating, advocating, supporting, and evaluating. An example of a limited classification system for stressors is illustrated by the following four categories: (1) deprivation, (2) excess, (3) change, and (4) intolerance.

Copyright © 1980 by Betty Neuman. Revised 1987 by Betty Neuman. Reprinted by permission.

Table 18-2
The Neuman Nursing Process Format

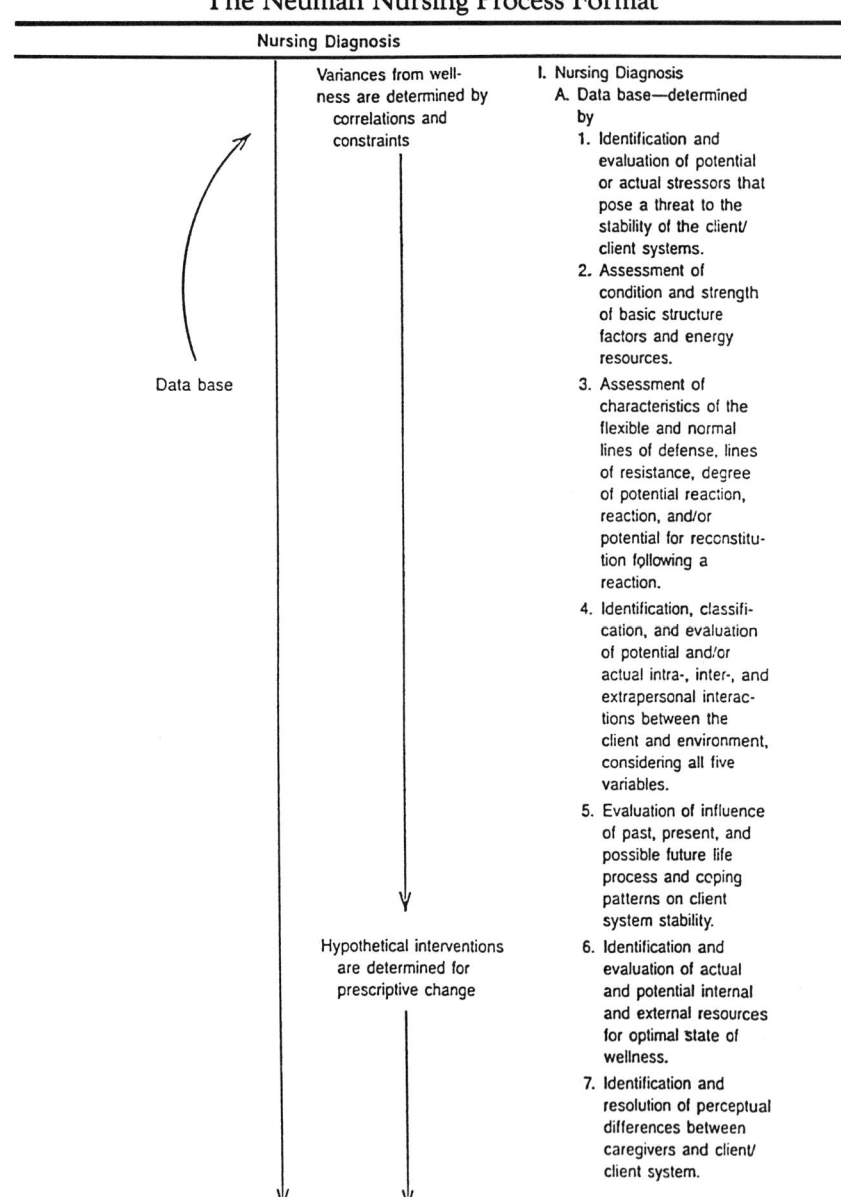

Nursing Diagnosis

Data base	Variances from wellness are determined by correlations and constraints ↓ Hypothetical interventions are determined for prescriptive change ↓	I. Nursing Diagnosis A. Data base—determined by 　1. Identification and evaluation of potential or actual stressors that pose a threat to the stability of the client/client systems. 　2. Assessment of condition and strength of basic structure factors and energy resources. 　3. Assessment of characteristics of the flexible and normal lines of defense, lines of resistance, degree of potential reaction, reaction, and/or potential for reconstitution following a reaction. 　4. Identification, classification, and evaluation of potential and/or actual intra-, inter-, and extrapersonal interactions between the client and environment, considering all five variables. 　5. Evaluation of influence of past, present, and possible future life process and coping patterns on client system stability. 　6. Identification and evaluation of actual and potential internal and external resources for optimal state of wellness. 　7. Identification and resolution of perceptual differences between caregivers and client/client system.

Copyright © 1980 by Betty Neuman. Revised 1987 by Betty Neuman. Reprinted by permission.

Table 18-2 (Continued)

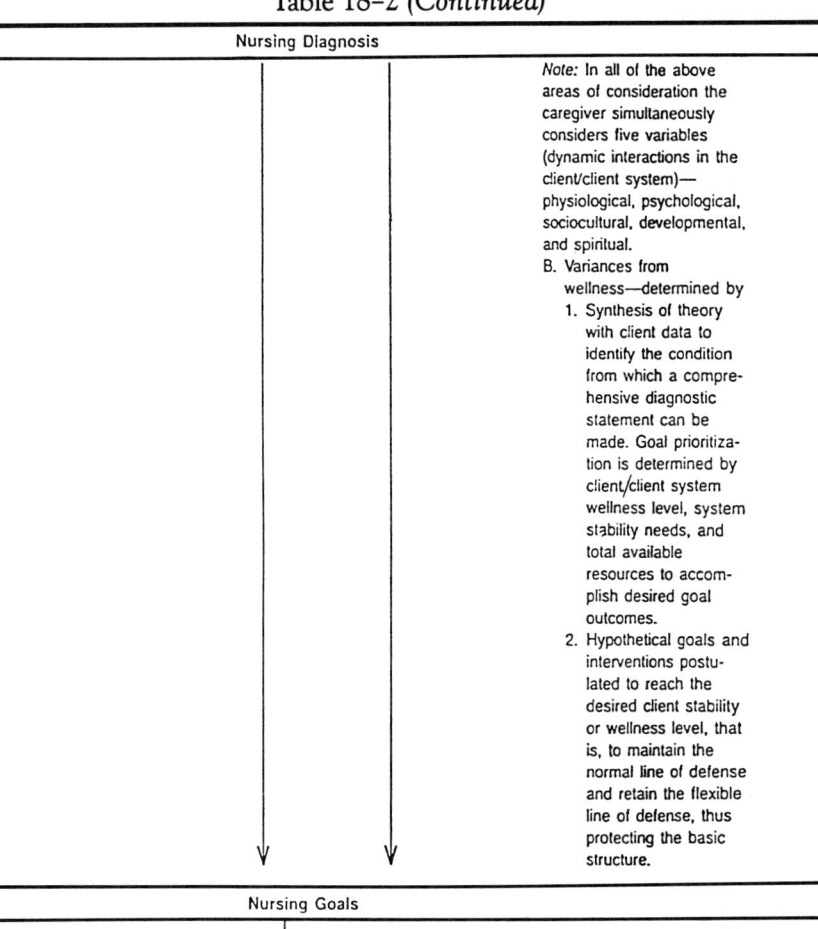

Nursing Diagnosis

Note: In all of the above areas of consideration the caregiver simultaneously considers five variables (dynamic interactions in the client/client system)—physiological, psychological, sociocultural, developmental, and spiritual.

B. Variances from wellness—determined by
  1. Synthesis of theory with client data to identify the condition from which a comprehensive diagnostic statement can be made. Goal prioritization is determined by client/client system wellness level, system stability needs, and total available resources to accomplish desired goal outcomes.
  2. Hypothetical goals and interventions postulated to reach the desired client stability or wellness level, that is, to maintain the normal line of defense and retain the flexible line of defense, thus protecting the basic structure.

Nursing Goals

Caregiver-client/client system negotiation for prescriptive change

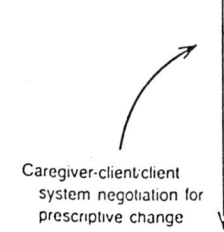

Caregiver intervention strategies negotiated to retain, attain, and maintain client/client system stability

II. Nursing goals—determined by
  A. Negotiations with the client for desired prescriptive change or goal outcomes to correct variances from wellness, based on classified needs and resources identified in the nursing diagnosis.
  B. Appropriate prevention as intervention strategies are negotiated with the client

continued

Table 18-2 (Continued)

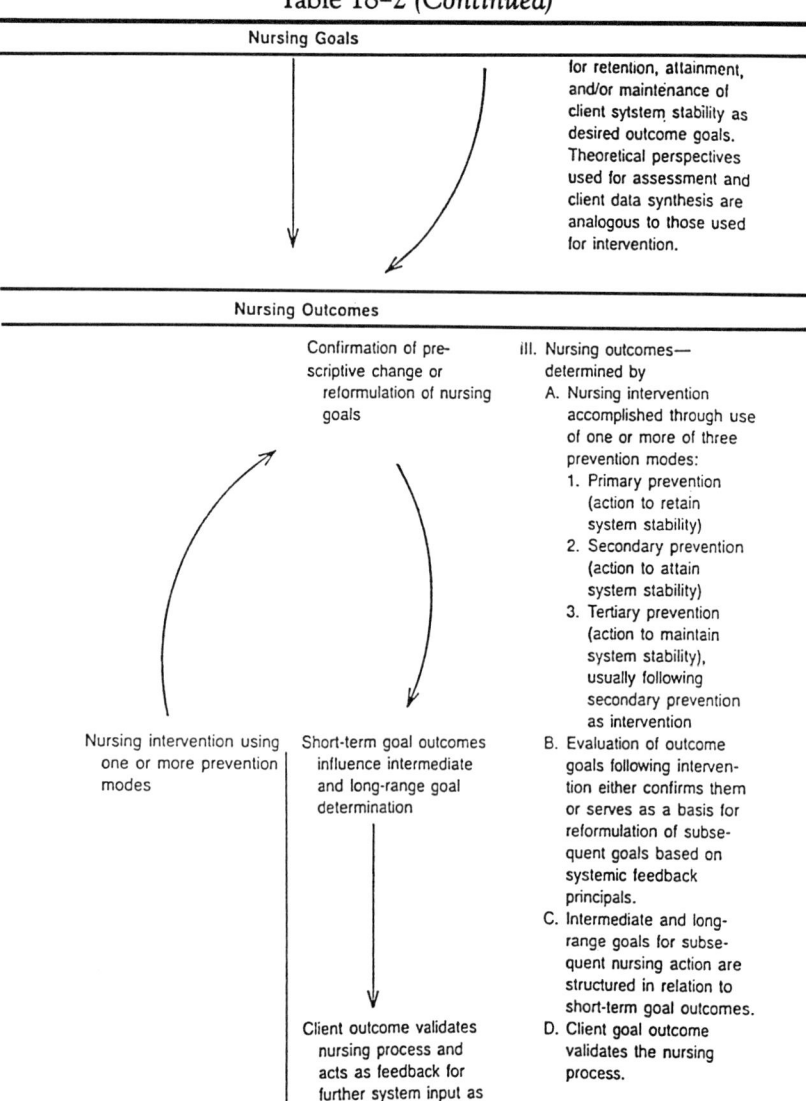

Nursing Goals

for retention, attainment, and/or maintenance of client sytstem stability as desired outcome goals. Theoretical perspectives used for assessment and client data synthesis are analogous to those used for intervention.

Nursing Outcomes

Confirmation of prescriptive change or reformulation of nursing goals

Nursing intervention using one or more prevention modes

Short-term goal outcomes influence intermediate and long-range goal determination

Client outcome validates nursing process and acts as feedback for further system input as required

III. Nursing outcomes—determined by
  A. Nursing intervention accomplished through use of one or more of three prevention modes:
    1. Primary prevention (action to retain system stability)
    2. Secondary prevention (action to attain system stability)
    3. Tertiary prevention (action to maintain system stability), usually following secondary prevention as intervention
  B. Evaluation of outcome goals following intervention either confirms them or serves as a basis for reformulation of subsequent goals based on systemic feedback principals.
  C. Intermediate and long-range goals for subsequent nursing action are structured in relation to short-term goal outcomes.
  D. Client goal outcome validates the nursing process.

WELLNESS WITHIN THE NEUMAN SYSTEMS PERSPECTIVE

Holism in the Neuman Systems Model is concerned with the entire client system in interaction with the internal and external environment. The entire system is considered to be larger than the sum of its parts. It is an open system in that input and output of the five variables, as parts of the system, interrelate with environmental stressors creating a multidimensional, comprehensive systemic view and holistic approach for caregivers.

The outer boundary of the system contains interacting parts and must be so defined. This boundary is illustrated by the flexible line of defense that protects the normal line of defense. The usual or normal wellness level is determined through assessment of the usual health status that has evolved as a consequence of the system's interacting part's adjustment or failure to adjust to stressors over time. Deviance from wellness is determined using the usual status of the normal line of defense as a standard against which to assess the degree of reduced wellness. *Wellness* within the system perspective is a broad concept with infinite complexities and possibilities, making it imperative that the normal line of defense be used as a standard for establishing the usual wellness condition against which to measure degrees of variance or deviance. Thus, the dynamic concept of wellness is best understood within the systems perspective. Through conceptualizing in this manner, it becomes possible to move from system structural concerns to functional or interactive relationships occurring among the parts which ideally accomplish system stability.

The system itself, then, becomes the structure within which its parts function through processes of interactions, interrelationships, and interdependencies. The constant dynamic motion or movement inherent within the parts has the goal of keeping the system as a structure stable. Ideally, movement of the system parts is toward a higher level of differentiation, function, and wellness while system structural integrity is maintained. Because of the circularity of the dynamic nature of systemic change, as it takes place within and surrounding the client, wellness can be logically viewed as being on a *continuum of wellness to illness* representing the system's energy level. Each successive encounter between the client's five-variable system and environmental stressors has the predictable outcome of either enhancing or diminishing system function and ultimately affecting the wellness level. Ideally, output or product of these cyclical processes acts as valuable feedback for input, further enhancing the system. In this manner, the quality of the interacting parts is supported with the ultimate goal of facilitating the highest possible degree of wellness or client system stability through purposeful energy conservation.

Since the concept of wellness within the systemic perspective has major implications for clients and caregivers for optimizing client wellness, the following cognitive factors (psychological variables) are considered, though not conclusively, as being relevant to effective individual client system coping and energy conservation:

- life-style (needs, expectations, motivation, and goals);
- personality type (psychodynamic factors); and
- coping ability (use of available resources).

For a group system, the following elements are considered relevant:

- purpose (needs and goals);
- roles/rules (interaction patterns); and
- resources (availability and use).

It is important to establish and monitor healthy coping patterns within the defined system parts to minimize the effects of stress and maximize the wellness level through energy conservation. Through healthy coping, available energy is both released and generated enhancing the client wellness level. Expected outcomes are improved quality care and optimal client system stability or wellness level.

Wellness is considered to be a more consolidated state and of a higher qualitative degree than is health as a concept. If all clients, ideally, were to choose wellness as their goal, the healing quality of caring would be reflected in the degree of understanding and skill demonstrated by the caregiver—one who truly understands the nature, needs, and possibilities of the system through highly motivated, knowledgeable, sensitive commitment and involvement.

THE MODEL AS A GUIDE FOR ACUTE AND CRITICAL CARE

Acute and critical care are similar in that clients receive relatively short-term care. Using the Neuman Systems Model, the major goal for nursing in both short- and long-term care is system stability. Because of the historic dearth of information on short-term often intensive care situations, the following abstracted or generic use of the model has been outlined to facilitate improved client care.

When the Neuman Model is used, the five client system variables should be assessed as to both existing strengths and weaknesses to establish the overall health condition. A first consideration should be the determination of a generic normal line of defense (inclusive of the five variables) peculiar to a specific class of clients and to the following developmental age ranges: four to 12, 12 to 17, 17 to 34, 35 to 65, and over 65.

This process would establish a generic form or level of wellness within the normal health range for the various stages of growth and development, against which deviance from wellness could be more accurately assessed in acute care situations. For example, in considering the progressively disabled schizophrenic client, a predetermined "generic" reduced wellness level or norm would be established to represent the usual health condition. One factor in such a predetermination might be that hypo- or hypersensitivity, with anxiety, lies at the base of all mental illness as a stressor.

The following ideas are proposed for use in any acute or short-term care situation in lieu of a more lengthy and detailed nursing process. In variable assessment, I have found the following to be true:

- Physiological—Strengths and impairments become behaviorally observable and known through laboratory findings.

- Psychological—Major focus behaviorally would be related to either withdrawal or intrusiveness.
- Sociocultural—Learned values act as either facilitating or impeding factors.
- Spiritual—The belief system acts as a positive resource or as a deficit.

The nature of environmental stressors is determined and considered in terms of the severity of client reaction or potential reaction. Stressors are considered unmet needs related to one or more of the five variables. Client behaviors may either increase or decrease the stress level. For example, socialization versus isolation relates to compliance and use of available resources, either of which may be influenced by knowledge factors and locus of control.

Examples of environmental stressors are the following:

- Intrapersonal—Cognitive ability, thoughts, and feelings
- Interpersonal—Close proximity interactions with others including caregivers.
- Extrapersonal—Quality of surroundings, more distal environment. For example, caregiver shortage, financial deficit, and inadequate support system.

A comprehensive nursing assessment is essential to the establishment of a relevant nursing diagnosis, goal planning, and appropriate nursing actions at the secondary prevention or treatment level, especially in short term and/or acute care situations. Simultaneous consideration of primary and tertiary aspects of preventive care defines the quality of holistic nursing.

Using this author's views for holistic short-term care assessment (following careful evaluation of available resources including time), it is both logical and possible to set care priorities on (1) optimal client system stability; (2) support of activities of daily living; and (3) care compliance; within short-term, acute, and critical care situations.

Thus, generic use of the Neuman Model lies within the purvue of its original intent and purpose, as the caregiver acts in the client's best interest to provide optimal holistic care within limited care situations. Table 18-3 is provided as a guide for program planning.

Table 18-3
Neuman Systems Model Philosophic Statements

Client	Environment	Health	Nursing
The client is an open system that interacts with the environment in order to promote harmony and balance between the internal and external environment. The client is a composite of physiologic, psychologic, sociocultural, developmental, and spiritual variables that are viewed as parts of the whole. Ideally the client as a system adjusts successfully to internal and external environmental stressors retaining the normal wellness level or system stability.	Environment contains both internal and external stressors and resistance factors. Lines of resistance in the client (internal and external resources) are activated to combat potential or actual stressor reactions. The flexible line of defense protects the normal line of defense or usual wellness condition while the lines of resistance protect the basic structure and support return to wellness. Stressors are considered neutral; client encounter determines either a beneficial or noxious outcome.	Health represents a usual dynamic stability state of the normal line of defense. A reaction to stressors is caused as the normal line of defense is penetrated, causing illness symptoms. The client's position on his or her own wellness-illness continuum is related to the amount of available energy stored and/or used by the system in retaining, attaining, and maintaining system stability.	Nursing is concerned with reduction of potential or actual stressor reaction through use of primary, secondary, or tertiary prevention as intervention to retain, attain, and maintain an optimal wellness level. The goal of nursing is optimal client system stability or wellness. Perceptual distortions between client and nurse, as well as goal plans, are mutually negotiated and resolved.

THE FUTURE OF THE MODEL

Features of the Neuman Systems Model most valued since its development are its comprehensive, flexible, and holistic systemic nature. The Neuman Model encompasses all nursing phenomena, and its social utility is well established in nursing education, administration, practice, and research. It is adapting well to other cultures.

The model is broadly based and congruent with newer health mandates of primary prevention of potential health problems. It considers client perception and mutual goal setting with clients. It has been successfully used in a wide variety of curricular patterns for student learning and practice areas to meet specific needs for individuals, aggregate groups, and the community. Its systemic base and concepts will continue their relevancy by incorporating future changes occurring in nursing.

Specific advantages of using the model, as stated by various nurses, are summarized as follows:

> The terminology is familiar and easily understood by both clients and caregivers. Its concepts can be taught as both content and process. It adapts well to all nursing phenomena across cultural boundaries. It has the flexibility to incorporate current and future trends in the field, which assures its continued utility and relevancy. The model clearly provides the systemic perspective and tools required for holistic nursing practice and theory development.

This author's (Neuman, 1990) perspectives on particular advantages of using a holistic systems-based model for nursing education and practice are conceptualized in the following statements. There is

- continuing socialization away from the medical model while the necessary component of illness treatment is retained;
- conceptualization of nursing as a maturing profession with unlimited boundaries for creativity in programming for quality nursing education and client care;

- an increasing number of comprehensive and holistic structures for organization of autonomous client health services;
- foundational relevance for incorporation of newer information in keeping with changing health mandates;
- need for consistent organization tools for reducing nursing education and service fragmentation; and
- guidance for nursing research and theory development.

In presenting the Neuman Systems Model, a comprehensive systemic view of nursing has been provided. Newer conceptualizations include the (Neuman, 1989) created-environment and energy relationship as a concept to optimize client wellness. The concept of wellness within the systems perspective (Neuman, 1990) is developed to facilitate the optimal wellness condition through consideration of coping ability and energy conservation. These concepts and a generic plan (Neuman, 1990) set forth for use of the model in short-term, acute, and intensive care situations will enhance future use of the model.

REFERENCES

Neuman, B. (1989). *The Neuman Systems Model.* Norwalk, CT: Appleton & Lange.

Neuman, B. (1990, April). *Using Nursing Theory in Clinical Practice.* Paper presented at the second Florida Nursing Theorist Conference, Miami, FL.

19

Implementation of the Neuman Systems Model in an Acute Care Nursing Department

Margaret M. Moynihan

This chapter will describe the implementation of the Neuman Systems Model of Nursing as the practice framework for nursing in an acute-care institution. I will first describe the practice setting and then the processes involved in writing a nursing philosophy, choosing the Neuman model as a theoretical base for practice, and implementing this model into practice. I will then present our current three-year plan.

When I joined the nursing management team in June 1985, Mount Sinai Hospital was a 359-bed acute-care inner city hospital. The nursing care delivery system, primary nursing, had been in place for several years. There was a clinical ladder system of advancement in place for the staff nurses. We had affiliating diploma, associate, baccalaureate, and master's degree students using our clinical resources for practical experience. The nursing administration was very supportive of individuals advancing their educational goals. About 70 percent of the nursing staff were professionals, and there was a good blend of experienced and inexperienced nurses. There was a readiness at Mount Sinai to challenge new areas of professional practice.

A one-year project of the nursing department began in 1986 and culminated in the identification of Mount Sinai nurses' beliefs concerning person, environment, health, and nursing. After developing and disseminating a nursing philosophy statement, we identified Neuman's Systems Model (1982) for implementation into practice at Mount Sinai.

PHILOSOPHY IDENTIFICATION

Nursing Management believed that active participation on the part of both management and staff was needed for acceptance of any philosophy statement. To facilitate a joint project, an existing staff advisory committee became the staff representative. A nursing faculty consultant joined the combined staff advisory/management group to help facilitate the process by providing assistance in relating nursing theory and philosophy, and in understanding the process of theory development.

During the planning process, the combined staff/management committee developed a survey that used both qualitative and quantitative approaches to draw out the respondents' philosophies. Items surveyed were beliefs about person, health, environment, illness, and nursing. A short forced-choice form was sent to all nurses. A more detailed, open ended questionnaire was sent to 100 nurses at random. Questionnaires were returned and tabulated.

Elements clearly identified by the nurses as being important to include in our philosophy statement were:

1. appreciation for the uniqueness of the person;
2. inclusion of variables that concern the physical, psychological, and spiritual dimensions of patient care;
3. appreciation for the client as a decision maker in the care/cure process;
4. a belief that the essence of nursing is caring;

5. recognition of the monitoring functions for medical interventions, and the independent and interdependent nursing interventions;
6. identification of a nursing goal to restore the patient to a state of dynamic equilibrium or support a dignified end to life;
7. identification of the target of nursing care as the patient, family, and/or significant other; and
8. a belief that the responsibility for the outcome of nursing care is shared by the patient and nurse.

Once the data were tabulated and a philosophy was drafted, it was circulated to the staff via their representatives. The philosophy was revised three times before it was finalized. We not only wanted all the nursing staff to embrace it, but we also wanted the rest of the institution to know that we had a unified statement of beliefs that was to be the foundation of the nursing department. We decided to report our activities to three of the most powerful committees in the hospital: the Medical-Executive committee, the Patient Care committee, and the Administrative committee. In doing so, we opened ourselves up to critique by other members of the hospital community. We received both supportive and nonsupportive comments. In particular, some non-nursing department heads commented that they felt left out of the survey. Once we had a written philosophy, we were able to distinguish between nursing department philosophy and hospital mission, which was a real issue within the institution at that time.

Once our philosophy project was implemented, we held education sessions for the staff, discussed it in orientation programs for new employees, and recognized the need for future planning to flow from the philosophy. It soon became obvious that the development of a philosophy was only a very first step. We now had to actualize the philosophy in daily practice.

IDENTIFICATION OF OUR NURSING MODEL

Our next goal was to identify how we would actualize the potential of the philosophy in daily practice. In answer, we planned to organize the daily practice of nursing around a nursing model appropriate for our philosophy. Several participants wanted to find a good fit with an already established model in order to be able to build upon an established base of knowledge, so as not to reinvent the wheel, but rather reach new heights of professional practice. Others were ready to develop "The Mount Sinai Model."

We chose to investigate the potential of what was published in the literature before we investigated the development of our own model. However, it was clear that if agreement could not be achieved with what was already published, then we were ready to challenge the development process.

Models per se were not new for many of our staff and managers. Each of our affiliating schools organized their curriculums around models, although not necessarily pure nursing models. Concepts about crisis and the nursing models of Nightingale and Rogers were three frameworks used by these schools to guide their curricula. Our management group had many master's students who were taking theory courses. The nursing administration was clearly vested in moving the department to a higher level of professional practice. The department had practiced a rather pure form of primary nursing for over ten years. Clinical levels of practice had been in place for staff advancement for eight years. There was a continuing goal to actualize department research projects around practice issues. There was a faculty practice in place with the University of Connecticut School of Nursing. The time was right!

With support from our faculty consultant, the staff/management committee identified what should exist in any model for practice, what our philosophy already defined for us, and what specific nursing models were in the literature. Our consultant did a literature search that identified three potential nursing models that appeared to be congruent with our philosophy: Roy's Adaptation Model (1984), Neuman's Systems Model, and Levine's Conservation Model (1973). The consultant prepared and presented a grid of the three models that compared how each represented person, environment, health, and nursing. Following a general discussion of each model, the committee decided it particularly wanted to investigate Roy's Adaptation Model and Neuman's Systems Model. Levine's terminology was thought to be unfamiliar to staff, especially considering what curriculum models had been used to organize their nursing education.

Subgroups within the staff/management committee were formed to prepare a debate around the pros and cons of each model for presentation to the committee and other interested staff and managers. The subgroups were to consider each model with regard to its compatibility with our philosophy and its ease of implementation. When all questions had been investigated, we sought consensus. This was achieved with the Neuman Systems Model. The missing piece for us in Neuman's model was the absence of the spiritual element. We added it to our model. We were very pleased to have this spiritual component added by Neuman (1989) in her revision. The whole process of choosing a model took six months to complete.

Identifying the nursing model was just the beginning. Implementation became viewed as an ominous process. In order to bring some reality and sanity into the process, we identified time frames for some goals. We knew we had to start with nursing assessment; we knew we wanted to have all units use the same model and assessment tool. We also had some Joint Commission on the Accreditation of Health Care Organizations (JCAHO) criteria to meet for 1989. We had to address changing issues because we now had a significant shortage of nursing professionals, primary nursing was much more difficult to implement as the staff-to-patient ratio increased, and the hospital declared financial jeopardy because of the unequal distribution of governmental payer patients versus insurance payers.

The agreed-upon central objective was to implement Neuman's model into everyday practice with the goal of showing how use of the model could make a difference in patient outcomes, nursing practice, and management ability to keep the hospital afloat. We began with nursing assessment, dividing the staff/management committee into two. One subgroup would be responsible for designing a self-study booklet on the Neuman Systems Model. The second group undertook the task of developing a new assessment tool. The two subgroups brought back information to the staff/management group for final approval. Staff involvement was seen as essential for any change to occur. Terminology had to be kept simple. There needed to be direct relatedness of the book and the assessment tool to the philosophy. The assessment tool needed to provide avenues for interdisciplinary work. The focus of the tool had to be on the patients and their responses. Generating patient outcomes related to quality assurance was the defined target. The nursing assessment tool had to be easy to use; increase the documentation of psychosocial, patient teaching, and discharge planning data; and lead to a nursing care plan that would be a permanent part of the patient record.

ASSESSMENT TOOL DEVELOPMENT

We began by asking nurses to identify assessment data they felt was essential to collect on admission in order to make the best possible initial nursing diagnosis. At the same time, the subgroup responsible for developing an assessment tool was exploring how to organize these data in Neuman's framework. Our attention shifted from assessing the five person variables (physiological, psychological, sociocultural, developmental, and spiritual) in each environmental stressor area (intrapersonal, interpersonal, and extrapersonal) to a more streamlined approach of assigning each of the person variables to one of the three environmental stressor areas. This approach avoided duplication but increased the chance of missing data. The question was, what was the significance of these missing data? We asked nurses on each patient unit to assess three patients using this new approach. The feedback indicated that some areas needed a section for specialized assessment according to the function of the unit. Three units developed a one-page specialty assessment addition to the nursing assessment form. These units were Adolescent Psychiatry, Labor and Delivery, and Pediatrics.

We responded to the feedback that completing the assessment "takes too long," by developing a tool with forced-choice questions that could be answered with checks or short answers. Our old form had open ended questions organized around functional health categories. With the nursing shortage at Mount Sinai, we were seeing an increase of missing data. A forced-choice format helped us cope with this quality assurance problem.

Once the form was revised in response to staff feedback and approved by the various hospital committees, we chose the Geriatric Unit as the pilot area to test the form for one month. At this time, the institution as a whole was facing major changes because of increasing acuity, lack of staff, financial constraints, and increased competition for staff in the Hartford area. We respected change theory and chose not to continue rapidly to organize nursing practice around a nursing theory. Instead, we chose to continue defining terminology, discussing organization of data in the Neuman framework, and streamlining documentation. We focused on the upcoming JCAHO Survey, the integration of more nursing assistants into our staff, and the process of moving from development of an assessment tool to actual implementation on a unit. By choosing not to rapidly implement a nursing theory, but rather to use the terminology and define it within our written structure, we were able to control the rate of change at a manageable level. Following the pilot project, each nursing division was educated in the model and then implemented the new nursing assessment tool. This was accomplished with the usual irritability reflective of change by December 1988. The Quality Assurance committee took over monitoring compliance of use of the assessment tool on each unit. The nursing department as a team became vested in getting ready for JCAHO in September 1989.

DEVELOPMENT OF AN EDUCATIONAL BOOKLET

The subcommittee responsible for designing educational materials for the Neuman Systems Model decided on a self-directed learning module approach. The booklet begins with a brief discussion of conceptual models in general and discusses reasons for applying a nursing model to a practice setting. It then specifies the Neuman Model in terms of person, environment, health, and nursing. It discusses stressors in relation to the three levels of prevention. There is in-depth content on appropriate goals and interventions for each level of prevention. The booklet concludes with two case studies that demonstrate use of the Neuman Model in the nursing process. The final page is for comments to the author on the content utilization by the learner. Eventually, we may apply to offer continuing education credit to nurses who use the booklet as a self-study program. Feedback has been positive in that it's an easy booklet to use and provides an introduction to the Neuman Systems Model.

PATIENT OUTCOMES

One goal in developing the nursing assessment tool was to make a direct connection between assessment data collected, patient outcomes, and the quality assurance process. The area of fall risk is where we have achieved our best results to date. Upon admission, each patient is assessed for the presence of stressors that would put him or her at risk for a fall. If the patient is considered at risk for a fall, then the standard of care "potential for injury/fall risk" is implemented. While this is a nursing standard, it is designed to make all hospital employees aware of the fall potential of this patient on or off the unit. The unit-based Quality Assurance committee follows the incident reports for falls and can identify whether a patient was appropriately assessed on admission. Primary preventions can decrease the fall rate. This can potentially reduce institutional insurance rates because of an actual decrease in occurrence of falls.

Another example of increased documentation of quality assurance provided by implementation of the model is a nonspecific evaluation of the completion of each section of the nursing assessment tool. The goal of this evaluation is to reinforce basic Neuman terminology.

FORMAL EDUCATION

The time was right to develop and present a formal class describing the Neuman Systems Model in nursing practice. Objectives for the class encompassed all aspects of the model. This class is the first attempt we have made at a purely educational offering to describe the model. The plan was to offer the class five times in 1990.

January and March have passed and people have been slow to select this class. We have decided that it needs to be marketed in a different framework or maybe the content should be divided into smaller sessions with new titles.

On a more positive note, two unit-based quality assurance committees have requested consultation for the purpose of increasing their understanding of the model so they can better monitor use of the assessment tool. This may be a clue that small group work related to standards will be the vehicle to provide education in the model.

Our shared governance structure has also been a vehicle for education. Members of each council within the structure have had a one-hour presentation on the model that included discussion of specific areas of their critical functions that need to be integrated with Neuman's model. These representatives report back to their respective constituency. In this way, the language of the Neuman Model is spreading.

THE FUTURE

In January 1990, we approved our next three-year Nursing Department Plan. The plan was developed with 12 staff nurse representatives. This is truly a Nursing Department (management and staff) plan. A surveillance committee was established to meet quarterly to monitor the plan's progress. Again, this is shared work.

The Neuman implementation plan includes the following time line:

- January 1990–1991 —Offer five formal Neuman classes in January, March, May, September, and November.

  —Continue to stress Neuman terminology in our discussion of nursing process.

  —Continue to develop quality assurance monitors and standards of care.

- May 1990 — Present a poster session on the implementation of the Neuman Systems Model in practice at the annual meeting of the American Organization of Nurse Executives.
- June 1990 — Begin to formulate a research proposal that addresses the assumptions of the model. Does using the Neuman model in a practice setting make a difference in patient outcomes? Our standards of care on stressors which may lead to falls could be a part of this research study.
- October 1990 — Attend Neuman's symposium.
- January 1991 — Conduct five-year evaluation of original philosophy assumptions (tool already developed).
  — Evaluate formal education process.
  — Begin implementation of research project.
- September 1991 — Publish research results.
  — Develop a liaison with faculty and graduate students to do some appropriate studies.
- January 1992 — Evaluate all projects.
  — Develop next three-year plan, if appropriate.

Mount Sinai as an institution has many challenges ahead. In order to facilitate financial equilibrium, we are processing an agreement for merger with another hospital. The impact this will have on the Nursing Department is uncertain. We have our goals set, however, understanding that time lines may change, people may change, the organization will change, but that nursing service has become sophisticated enough to recognize that good patient care doesn't just happen. There must be a philosophical foundation of beliefs that dictate an organizational process, preferably a nursing theory, that provides the basic framework for practice. It's only then that we can logically test our reality to see how significant are nursing's contributions to patient outcomes.

REFERENCES

Levine, M. E. (1973). *Introduction to clinical nursing.* (2nd ed.). Philadelphia: F.A. Davis.

Neuman, B. (1982). *The Neuman Systems Model.* Norwalk, CT: Appleton-Century-Crofts.

Neuman, B. (1989). *The Neuman Systems Model.* Norwalk, CT: Appleton & Lange.

Roy, C. (1984). *Introduction to nursing: An adaptation model.* Englewood Cliffs, NJ: Prentice-Hall, Inc.

Part 9

Watson's Theory of Caring in Nursing

20

Transpersonal Caring: A Transcendent View of Person, Health, and Healing

M. Jean Watson

We are acutely aware of the fact that nursing is in dramatic transition and is already in the process of being redefined. Conferences such as this theory conference, combined with synergistic networks across the country, are helping to bring about what some are referring to as a revolution, a reformation, and a transformation in the human consciousness. Organizations such as the American Holistic Nursing Association and the National League for Nursing, the movement called the Curriculum Revolution, various specialty groups in nursing, feminist writers, and nursing theorists are all empowering themselves through their commitments and their changing consciousness to more fully actualize nursing and the human caring, healing, and health dimensions of nursing. All of us are seeking at some level, wherever we are, to bring about a new consciousness of what it means to be a nurse,

---

Note: This paper draws upon earlier work by Watson (1988), New Dimensions in Human Caring Theory, *Nursing Science Quarterly*, *1*(4), 175–181 and papers presented at Catholic University and Boston College.

to be caring. Thus, we are here to work toward a new social order whereby nursing and caring can exist or at least coexist along with the techno-cure order of today (Watson, 1990).

As pointed out in an earlier publication (Watson, 1988), nursing has some new options. Rather than having to stay within the same debate of fighting disease and death or postponing or denying or fearing death and disease, we have another moral course—if not ontological and scientific course—in positing the notion of caring-healing as a moral ideal and an end in and of itself (Gadow, 1985; Watson, 1988). Such thinking allows nursing theory to emerge as a forthright, authentic model that does not have to remain in conflict with the larger and more dominant ideology of the health care system. This model of caring-healing can accommodate some of the new world views and moral ideals that guide nursing actions.

While caring and traditional treatments can and perhaps must be present when curing is called for, certainly caring must be present when curing has failed, and death with dignity is the last result. Human caring is at the same time a place in which we as health professionals can, do, and must live even when—especially when no cure is possible—but also even when cure is possible (Gadow, 1988; Watson, 1988).

The caring framework I'm concerned with requires an expanded view of nursing, science, person, and health-illness. It concerns the following precepts: nursing in relation to transpersonal caring consciousness, science in relation to human science dimensions, person in relation to a transcendent view of human, and medical treatment and cure as secondary to health and healing.

Viewing nursing within a transpersonal caring-healing perspective attends to the human center and caring-healing consciousness of both the nurse and the one being cared for; it embraces both a physical embodiment as well as a metaphysical transcendent dimension of nursing and the human caring-healing process; it is concerned with preserving human dignity and restoring and preserving humanity in the fragmented, technological, medical cure-dominated systems.

A different framework, one related to the transpersonal human caring-healing framework is one that is centered around the concept of intersubjectivity. In this framework, acknowledging inseparable connections among persons and between person and nature is essential to the quest for an expanded ontology of personhood beyond person as object and beyond the person as separate from others and nature (Watson, 1989). This approach is particularly poignant when considering a nurse-run community-based caring model, such as the Denver Nursing Project in Human Caring, also known as the "Caring Center."

What exactly is involved with these transcendent intersubjective notions of *human care and caring?* I will try to explain as well as illustrate through art, metaphor, and poetry. My explanation will also incorporate some key underlying theoretical and scientific positions. The last part of this chapter will draw upon the metaphor of a hologram as a call for evolution to a higher consciousness as part of the changing nature of science. Such thinking offers a new ontology of person as well as a new ontology of caring-healing that affects our epistemologies, methodologies, nursing praxis, and ultimately our very view of reality. More specific application of these caring theory concepts are developed by Neil (1990) in the next chapter.

To capture the comprehensive and complex nature of caring, I'd like to begin with a poem that reflects the complex yet basic human intersubjective dynamic in a transpersonal caring moment between a nurse and Mr. Polanski, an elderly man living in a nursing home. Mr. Polanski could also be an abandoned, vulnerable person with AIDS. The poetry is a result of Marilyn Krysl's commissioned work as a Visiting Poet in the Center for Human Caring at the University of Colorado School of Nursing.

The work is entitled *Sunshine Acres Living Center.* This is an earlier version of the poem by the same title in Krysl's (1989) book *Midwife and Other Poems on Caring.* Poetry is one form of language that is often necessary to convey the depth of transpersonal caring that we otherwise have no way to communicate.

SUNSHINE ACRES LIVING CENTER[*]

The first thing you see up ahead is Mr.
Polanski, wedged in the
arched doorway, like he means absolutely

---

[*] Reprinted by permission of Marilyn Krysl and the Center for Human Caring, University of Colorado School of Nursing.

to stay there, he who shouldn't
be here in the first place, put in here
by mistake, courtesy of that grandson
who thinks he's a hotshot, and too busy raking in
the dough to take time for an old
man. If he had anyplace to go, you know he'd be out
instantly, if he had any
money. So he intends

to stay in that doorway, not missing
a thing, and waiting
for trouble. Which of course
will come. And could be
you—you're handy, you look
likely, you have

the authority. And you're
new here, another young
whippersnapper, doesn't know
ankle from elbow, but has been given
the keys. Well he's
ready, Polanski. So you go right
to him. *Mr. Polanski, good
morning*—you say it in Polish,
which you learned a little of
when you were little, and your grandmother taught you
a little song about lambs, frisking
in a pen, and you
danced a silly little dance with your grandmother
while the two of you
sang. So you sing it

for him, here in the dim, institutional
light of the hallway, light which even you find
insupportable, because at that moment
it reminds you of the light in the hallway
in the resthome where, when your grandmother
died, you weren't
there. So that you're also singing
to console yourself. And at the moment you pay her
this silly little tribute, Mr. Polanski
steps out of the doorway. He

who had set himself to
resist you, he who had made himself
a first, Mr. Polanski,
> contentious
> often combative
> and always inconsolable

hears that you know
the song. And he steps out
from the fortress of the
doorway, begins

to shuffle
and sing along.

HUMAN CARING THEORY APPLIED

This poetic work helps me to introduce two major aspects of caring. The first aspect has to do with the interconnected, intersubjective aspects of caring between the one caring and the one cared for. The second notion has to do with the possibility of a movement toward transcendence that can occur in a transpersonal caring moment.

In my 1985 work, I define human caring in nursing as a moral ideal, in the sense that the nurse carries (or perhaps should carry) a caring consciousness in mind during every nursing transaction, as an ideal that will help point the way toward certain human caring actions. While such an ideal will not dictate specific behaviors, it will direct the nurse toward certain actions, and not toward others.

In the moment with Mr. Polanski, the nurse was presented with an opportunity to decide how to be in that caring moment—what to do with that moment. Her caring consciousness guided her in one manner and not another. Indeed, it was her personal-subjective human dimensions that were brought to bear as she tapped into Mr. Polanski's lived world, and which resulted in an intersubjectivity in which the person of both was involved.

In transpersonal caring, the nurse enters into the lived experience of another person, and that person enters into the nurse's experience. The caring moment Mr. Polanski and the nurse composed was filled with energy[1]—as much energy subjectively, as if he had leapt from the doorway into the dance. Objectively, the movement may have seemed minimal, surely too small to count as a nursing intervention or a therapy. Only from the inner personal field perspective does the actual subjective and intersubjective vitality emerge until contact is made—and transpersonal caring occurs as one field.

If we focus only on obstinacy, immobilization, anger, and hostility, we ignore the intersubjective caring field possibilities of Mr. Polanski and the nurse making human contact in the present moment. The present that Mr. Polanski and the timid, but bold, nurse created was filled with energy and transcendent acts that moved to intersubjective cultural realms beyond, yet also occupying the moment, and allowed a human-to-human awakening. The nurse was able to see a little of Mr. Polanski in herself and vice versa.

The two individuals in the human caring situation presented are both in a process of being and becoming. Each brings with them to the relationship a unique life history and phenomenological field, and both are influenced by the nature of the transaction.

As Moustakas put it: "The opportunity to engage in genuine caring is a process of intuitive awareness, sensing and knowing, a recognition of the mystery, the awe, the capriciousness, the unpredictability of life, the possibility of the power of silence and of real dialogue with others in the deep moments of life . . . and indeed spiritual qualities of our energy interchange via the caring relationship" (Moustakas, 1977).

As Greene (1986) says, "it is only in our intersubjectivity, our coming together that we create social space for caring, for values literacy, where transformation can occur." This thinking reminds us and returns us to the power of, if not reverence and regard for, what I call the sacred space that each caring occasion potentially contains, be it between patient and nurse or student and teacher (Watson, 1989).

Krysl describes the higher energy dimensions of transpersonal caring this way:

---

[1] These ideas were influenced by S. Gadow, 1988.

Caring for others takes place, so to speak, in the metaphysical realm. We cannot "see" this realm, but we experience it. Over and over I watched the caregiver and the person accepting care as they came to constitute one wholeness. When two of us enter into each other this way, willingly and receptively, transformation takes place. The gestalt of our separate beings loosens and vibrates. The material of our being and becoming begins to flow. We experience ourselves and each other as elemental substance. We experience the living field of our interconnectedness. And we are filled with energy, a living material, palpable, substantial. This energy is nearly visible in the air around us. It is as though we give off light.

These moments of transcendence are fascinating. They occurred again and again, each time flowering forth, a moment of intense energy, of very material presence. I felt I was witnessing the invisible made substance. I was witnessing the spirit made flesh. (Krysl, 1989).

HOLOGRAPHIC SCIENCE METAPHOR[2]

In the western world we try to titrate out human caring, as well as AIDS, for example. They are both what Benner (1987) suggests are personal and cultural embarrassments. If we could, we would sometimes slip care under the door and do likewise with those who are the most vulnerable—slip them out of the mainstream of science and society.

So how are we to understand changing human conditions, when medical science and technology do not solve the problem, or even when they offer some solutions, but also other consequences?

One science paradigm that offers a metaphorical model for some of the elusive concepts for caring-healing consciousness and human science is commonly referred to as the holographic paradigm. This perspective offers a view of wholeness in each of the related parts. Contemporary nursing theories (Newman, 1986; Parse, 1981; Rogers, 1970) accommodate the holographic perspective by defining human beings as energy fields, open systems

---
[2] This section draws upon Watson, 1988.

engaged in continual energy exchange with the environment, centers of energy, patterns of consciousness, and so on (Watson, 1988).

Because energy fields and patterns of consciousness are nonphysical phenomena, they are viewed as less real than a science of cells or the concept of physical causation. However, higher order concepts such as transpersonal caring-healing processes and caring field call for an expanded science model. As Moccia (1988) points out, fundamental issues related to ontologies, epistemologies, values, and intentions are now being questioned, clarified, and debated to address future directions for nursing science.

Regardless of one's theoretical inclinations, there is the continual need to search the traditional models of health and illness and acknowledge that they are inadequate for the lived caring-healing processes nurses experience in transpersonal caring moments. Just as poetry helps us to see the higher level dimensions of nursing, the metaphor of a hologram provides a new science model as well as a new gestalt for viewing the caring-healing transpersonal field.

Some of my earlier work presents some basic holographic principles applied to transpersonal caring:

- The whole caring-healing consciousness is contained in a single caring moment.
- The one caring-healing and the one-being-cared-for-healed are interconnected; caring and healing are connected to other humans, the environment, and to the higher energy of the universe.
- Human caring-healing (or noncaring-nonhealing) consciousness of the nurse is communicated to the one being cared for.
- Caring-healing consciousness is spatially extended; such consciousness exists through space.
- Caring-healing consciousness is temporally extended; such consciousness exists through time.
- Caring-healing consciousness is dominant over physical illness and treatment. (Adapted from Watson, 1988)

Such thinking can perhaps help us grasp a new view of caring and healing that ultimately calls for a new view and a new ontology of person that goes beyond the body physical and incorporates transcendence and evolving consciousness.

CARING IN ART

Alex Grey's art slide collection "The Sacred Mirror" helps us to visually, aesthetically, and artistically glimpse some of these notions of spiritual energy, higher consciousness, and caring-healing consciousness, all of which are so commanding in the latest thinking in science. As Teilhard de Chardin (1959) put it: "An interpretation of the universe remains unsatisfactory unless it covers the mind and the consciousness as well as the matter. The true physics is that which will one day achieve the inclusion of man (woman) in wholeness in a coherent picture of the world."

The art slides shown at the conference help to convey some of the beauty, mystery, and wonder of the human body and higher energy connections, suggesting new meaning of human-environment and our connectedness with a broader universe. The following art slides were shown:

1. Material World
2. Skeletal System
3. Nervous System
4. Cardiovascular System
5. Lymphatic System
6. Viscera
7. Muscular System
8. Caucasian Female
9. Caucasian Male
10. Black Female
11. Black Male
12. Oriental Female
13. Oriental Male
14. Life Energy System
15. Psychic Energy System
16. Spiritual Energy System
17. Universal Mind Lattice
18. Buddha of all Compassion
19. Christ
20. Spiritual World (Godhead)
21. Void/Clear Light

Perhaps we are evolving toward Teilhard's "Omega Point" (Teilhard, 1959) and can now acknowledge that there is a unity of consciousness and matter. Perhaps we are emerging with experience and through our evolution into a higher integration of spirituality and the material/physical world, resulting in a new ontology of person, caring, and healing possibilities. We can perhaps move toward what Newman (1986) calls an integrative functioning in our science, can now shift to the notion of consciousness and transcendence as context. This evolution, however, leads to new responsibilities as nurses and health professionals. This perspective is beyond the body physical. This thinking is congruent with the latest work of Larry Dossey (1990), *Recovering the Soul,* and Gary Zukav (1990), *The Seat of the Soul.*

We must continue our search to find new language and methods to capture the new ontology and its expanded, evolving consciousness and concept of soul, but now with a fresh, new, integrative higher consciousness view of transpersonal caring and healing. Thus, biomedical science and medical cure can be seen as only one component of nursing and caring science. We can now appreciate one last poetic work by Krysl from the Center for Human Caring—a work associated with human touch that transcends the body physical and can in turn touch the human heart, mind, and soul. It is entitled *Skin* and is an earlier version of the poem of the same title in *Midwife and Other Poems on Caring* (Krysl, 1989).

SKIN[*]

Because skin is the first organ
    to form in the womb, and first things
    are of first importance.

Because skin is the largest
    organ—an adult's, stretched out, weighs
    six pounds covers eighteen square feet
    and so there is more of it to attend to
    than anything else

Because the skin's resilience
    can only be experienced

Because it feels superior by far
    to silk or challis

    and in addition is lovely
    to look at, the body's

---

[*] Reprinted by permission of Marilyn Krysl and the Center for Human Caring, University of Colorado School of Nursing.

    haute couture: nothing by Cardin
    comes close to it

Because it's the organ with which we experience wind,
    which most loves water,
    and with which we take sunlight inside us

because, because, because, because,
    and for all these good reasons

hurry out and touch someone now!

    Delay in this matter
    is not
    a good idea, you
    delayed too long
    already, your suffering brothers and sisters
    are waiting, you can hardly
    expect them to wait much
    longer, and remember
    when you touch the skin of another person
    they feel better, and you feel
    stronger

because the skin of another person
gives off a chemical

which makes you, and them,
    feel better
    more alert
    more cheerful
    and willing to take changes
    more open to new experience
    more generally obstreperously intent

    on securing the greatest good
    for everybody
    and more likely to say NO to the MX
    and YES to the levy for the public schools.

Remember
it's the organ
through which we take in
the light we give out

REFERENCES

Dossey, L. (1990). *Recovering the soul*. New York: Bantam Books.

Gadow, S. (1985). Nurse and patient: The caring relationship. In A. H. Bishop and J. R. Scudder (Eds.). *Caring, curing, coping* (pp. 31–43). Tuscaloosa, AL: University of Alabama Press.

Gadow, S. (1988). Covenant without cure: Letting go and holding on in chronic illness. In J. Watson and M. A. Ray (Eds.). *The ethics of care and the ethics of cure: Synthesis in chronicity* (pp. 5–14). New York: National League for Nursing.

Greene, M. (1986). Toward possibility: Expanding the range of literacy. *English Education, 18,* 231–243.

Krysl, M. (1989). *Midwife and other poems on caring*. New York: National League for Nursing.

Moccia, P. (1988). A critique of promise: Beyond the methods debate. *Advances in Nursing Science, 10*(4), 1–9.

Moustakas, C. F. (1977). *Creative life*. New York: Van Nostrand, Reinhold.

Newman, M. (1986). *Health as an expanding consciousness*. St. Louis, MO: C. V. Mosby.

Parse, R. (1981). *Man-living-health: A theory of nursing*. New York: John Wiley & Sons.

Rogers, M. (1970). *An introduction to the theoretical basis of nursing*. Philadelphia, PA: Davis.

Teilhard de Chardin, P. (1959). *The phenomenon of man*. New York: Harper & Brothers Publishers.

Watson, J. (1988). *Nursing: Human science and human care*. New York: National League for Nursing.

Watson, J. (1988). New dimensions of human caring theory. *Nursing Science Quarterly, 1*(4), 175–181.

Watson, J. (1989). Human caring and suffering: A subjective model for health sciences. In R. Taylor and J. Watson (Eds.). *They shall not hurt* (pp. 125–135). Boulder, CO: University Press of Colorado.

Watson, J. (1990). The moral failure of the patriarchy. *Nursing Outlook, 38*(2), 62–66.

Zukav, G. (1990). *The seat of the soul*. New York: Fireside Publications.

21

Watson's Theory of Caring in Nursing: The Rainbow of and for People Living with AIDS

Ruth M. Neil

In "Nursing on the Caring Edge" (Watson, 1987), several metaphors are offered to communicate the essence of nursing and its role in society. D.H. Lawrence's work *The Rainbow* is cited with emphasis on its reference to "the broken end of the arc."

In Watson's interpretation, medical science, technology, and the emphasis on cure are responsible for "the broken end of the arc" in the arena of human health and healing. "Whereas curative factors aim at *curing* the patient of disease, *'carative'* factors aim at the *caring process* that helps the person attain (or maintain) health or die a peaceful death" (Watson, 1985a).

Additionally, the broken arc can be seen when a single human life is broken by diagnosis with a fatal illness, especially when the person is young and even more especially when the illness itself invokes fear and stigma. AIDS, as a major disease in contemporary society, is such an illness. In the United States, over 122,000 cases have been reported since 1982 and between 1.5 million and 2 million people are estimated to carry the virus. The Centers for

Disease Control (CDC) predict that there will be up to 225,000 cases of AIDS in the United States by 1993 (Department of Health and Human Services, 1990). The caring offered by nursing holds up the broken arc and helps to capture the full spectrum of the rainbow, whether that rainbow represents the whole area of health care delivery or an individual human life.

METAPHORS AND AIDS

Viney (1983) reported that one important reality is what people imagine it to be. "This is as important for people dealing with illness as it is for people dealing with other events. It is the images of illness which people build up which affect how they act when illness becomes an important aspect of their own experience." " . . . the most important reality may not be the reality of the physical world but the reality which we create when we interpret the information we have about that world . . . it is only our images of illness that can be known to us, not the illnesses themselves . . . ."

As has been true of other devastating diseases, numerous authors have suggested images or metaphors for AIDS. In an article in a recent issue of *Medical Humanities Review* (Jones, 1990), the most common of these were identified as the military metaphor (with the body as the battleground); AIDS as pollution, contamination, or apocalypse; and AIDS as the plague.

The plague itself was used metaphorically (to represent interpersonal inhumanity) in Camus's novel (1972) of that title. In his reflective summary of his experiences caring for people dying of the plague, Dr. Rieux, Camus's storyteller, "knew that the tale he had to tell could not be one of a final victory. It could be only the record of what had had to be done, and what assuredly would have to be done again in the never ending fight against terror and its relentless onslaughts, despite their personal afflictions, by all who, while unable to be saints but refusing to bow down to pestilences, strive their utmost to be healers."

In describing the persons who died from the plague, Rieux "deliberately (took) the victims' side and tried to share with his fellow citizens the only certitudes they had in common—love, exile, and suffering . . . there was not one of their anxieties in which he did not share, no predicament of theirs that was not his" (Camus, 1972). Camus, through his character, Dr. Rieux, was emphasizing the *common humanity of all persons,* both those needing care and those giving care. He was also referring to the inadequacy of grouping or labeling all the people who died from the plague as "the same." The individuality of people living with AIDS is just as true.

It is for this reason Jones (1990) suggested that first-person narratives written by persons living with AIDS might be more useful than metaphors or theories. Contrasts between two such narratives excerpted by Jones emphasize the individuality of the AIDS experience:

> The very friends who tell me how vigorous I look, how well I seem, are the first to assure me of the imminent medical breakthrough. What they don't seem to understand is, I used up all my optimism keeping my friend alive. Now that he's gone, the cup of my own health is neither half full nor half empty. Just half (Jones, 1990).

> I have to keep dreaming blue skies
>   confronting the darkened cloud,
>   building sand castles
>   withstanding the beating wave,
>   overcoming imminent ills
>   opposing the dreaded dragon,
>   concluding happy ever after
>   crowning the victorious end.*

Individuals expressing their innermost thoughts think and write in metaphors, just as do writers attempting to express universal ideas. The reason for including the first excerpt in this paper is the analogy between "just half" and the brokenness of the arc

---

* Reprinted from Howard, B. (1989). *Epitaphs for the living: Words and images in the time of AIDS.* Dallas: Southern Methodist University Press. Reprinted by permission.

described by Lawrence. The second excerpt is included because of its expression of natural phenomena and images of victory similar to the wholeness suggested by the rainbow.

Images or metaphors are not only important in our thinking about disease processes, but also in society's response and our response as professional nurses to persons living with the disease. "People who are ill (or the people caring for them) need not be overwhelmed by their images of illness, if they are aware of their own role in constructing them. To know that one chooses the world in which one lives is to control it" (Viney, 1983). Some persons living with AIDS have adopted totally different kinds of metaphors to describe their diagnosis, including "a gift," "an opportunity," or "an interesting challenge." It is useful in working with clients to discover which metaphors or images have meaning for them and to experiment with different metaphors to find those that are most health-enhancing.

THE DENVER NURSING PROJECT IN HUMAN CARING

In thinking of Jean Watson's philosophy and science of human caring as "holding up the arc," it should be remembered that the "raison d'être" of this or any nursing theory is the human person and his or her quality of life and health. Thus, a metaphoric description of human beings is presented to complete the context for caring at the Denver Nursing Project in Human Caring (DNPHC). The metaphoric description used at DNPHC is paraphrased from *Emmanuel's Book* (Rodegast & Stanton, 1987). When asked "What does a human being look like?", Emmanuel answers:

> When I see a soul, I see Light—crystalline, pure, expanded and very beautiful. When I see a human being, I see that very same soul often cramped, struggling beneath an overlay of various diminishing hues that cause the brilliance to remain entrapped in the more opaque auric qualities . . . When I view you with my love, I see that Light very much as you do when you view each other with love.

Emmanuel's voice continues to describe the meaning of all the colors and encourages reawakened vision in those hearing him. His closing words are *"I see you all as rainbows."*

Theoretical Basis for DNPHC

The nursing care of clients (which deserves first priority), the care of staff (both professional staff and volunteer staff), the educational endeavors with students who come to DNPHC, the interactions with nursing administrators from the affiliated institutions, and the interactions with benefactors and supporters of DNPHC are all based, as consciously as possible, on Jean Watson's treatises on human caring.

> The *Mission Statement* (1989) of DNPHC includes the following words: . . . health care is based on respect for each person and belief that health and well-being are multidimensional—including physical, emotional, mental, spiritual and social components. Every person is unique and has the right and responsibility to make informed choices concerning health. Each person also possesses the inner resources and strengths to meet health challenges. The DNPHC staff, through the establishment of authentic caring relationships with the clients, assist and encourage them in self-acceptance, self-love, and self-empowerment. The staff belief is that the healing process is fostered by the understanding, love, and concern of those who care.

Using the Theory with Clients

Watson's first work (1985a), describing "carative" factors as aspects of her theory of nursing, provides the format for initial assessment interviews, development of care plans, and charting on clinic records. Figure 21–1 is a sample of charting which demonstrates how nurses at DNPHC are encouraged to be ever conscious of Watson's theory.

The human caring process demonstrates respect for the individual humanness of both the client and the nurse in a caring relationship. This process is both holistic and existential. Watson

Figure 21-1
Charting at the Denver Nursing Project
(Modification of SOAP (IE) Format)

A = assessment P = plan (care factor)
I = intervention E = evaluation

A. Walked into DNPHC appearing anxious and sad. States "My dog of 13 years was killed by a car last night and I haven't even been able to cry. What's wrong with me?"
P. Maintain sensitivity to self and others. Provide supportive environment. Encourage expression of feelings.
I. Discussed loss and grief and its cumulative effect. Reviewed with client recent losses related to his physical health/disease progression. Assured client that inability to grieve for his pet right now is not "abnormal."
E. (Five days later). Client returned describing an event at home during the weekend which triggered a "flood of tears" about his dog. Also asking for disease information more openly. Says he "feels more normal now."

wrote, " . . . the individuals . . . are both in a process of being and becoming. Both individuals bring with them to the relationship a unique life history and phenomenal field, and both are influenced and affected by the nature of the transaction, which in turn becomes part of the life history of each person. In this sense of a caring transaction, caring is a moral ideal, rather than an interpersonal technique and it entails a commitment to a particular end. The end is the protection, enhancement, and preservation of the person's humanity, which helps to restore inner harmony and potential healing" (Watson 1985b).

Caring theory is an excellent match for helping individuals who are HIV infected or have AIDS. AIDS represents a supreme existential and holistic challenge for persons living with the disease. Tillich (1952) described the existential anxieties experienced by humans as the anxiety of fate and death, the anxiety of emptiness and meaninglessness, and the anxiety of guilt and condemnation, which, if not faced and "lived through," result in despair. Despair is not health-inducing. Persons living with AIDS experience each of these anxieties and need to explore and find meaning in the realities of their illness. In the accepting and safe environment of DNPHC, the nurses—through authentic caring—assist clients in this process.

Using the Theory with Staff

Caring for the caregiver has received much recent emphasis as a necessity for prevention of turnover and burnout among professional caregivers. It is especially important for caregivers in a facility serving clients with terminal diagnoses. The environment of the Denver Nursing Project could seem to magnify the problem because of the nonclinical setting and the family-like relationships that exist among clients and staff.

In Benner's (1984) discussion of "involvement versus distance" in nurse-patient relationships, she hypothesized that by being *involved* with their clients (as occurs in the caring relationships at DNPHC), nurses are more fully able to draw on their own coping resources and the resources offered by the patient, the family, and the situation. Benner says, ". . . distancing techniques dimly protect nurses from the pain in the situation, but they also prevent them from taking advantage of the resources and possibilities that come through engagement and participation in the patients' and families' meanings and ways of coping."

Nurses at DNPHC consider the involvement with clients, often on an intimate emotional level, to be a privilege for the very reasons Benner identified. Sharing and grieving honestly with clients about the myriad losses AIDS induces fosters a climate in which the nurse can assist with realistic education, decision making, and problem solving. The clients and nurses work as partners in the process.

During regular staff support group meetings, frequent spontaneous one-on-one staff interactions, and meditation experiences, DNPHC nurses consider ". . . the tensions implicit in all human acts of care—the 'teach us to care and not to care' of T.S. Eliot's *Ash Wednesday"* (Campbell, 1984). Campbell, a theologian writing about the distinctions between professional and social caring, suggested that a way of understanding caring in nursing may be found by exploring the concept of companionship. Companionship describes closeness, implies movement and change, expresses mutuality, and requires commitment—but within defined limits. "It is a bodily presence which accompanies the other for a while. The image of the journey springs to mind when we think of the companion. Companionship arises often from a chance meeting and it is terminated when the joint purpose which keeps companions together no longer obtains. The good companion is someone who shares freely, but does not impose, allowing others to make their *own* journey" (Campbell, 1984). This image of companionship describes well the caring relationships between and among clients and staff at the Denver Nursing Project.

Research

In consciously applying Watson's theory of caring while interacting with clients at DNPHC, nurses have opportunity to contribute to the growth of caring knowledge. "Caring . . . elicits a transpersonal relationship where meaning becomes relational, expressive, and contextual . . . developing caring knowledge is risky business and hard work. It requires realistic commitment to self and others and creative knowledge construction, as well as compassionate motivation, emotional involvement and contextual competency and skills" (Watson, 1987).

Huch (1988) wrote that to practice nursing from an existing theory or framework requires intense study, time, and effort. Reasons for pursuing such an undertaking include the idea that theory-based practice structures nursing care in a consistent, systematized way and thus guides practice and facilitates evaluation. Additionally, theory-based practice is a way of pragmatically testing theories, leading to expansion of nursing's knowledge base.

Evidence from nurse-directed research supporting the efficacy of Watson's theory at DNPHC is not currently completed. The following expressions of client experience, however, provide testimony that the caring philosophy is being lived.

Clients discussing the Caring Center on the videotape "Theories at Work" included such remarks as, "People don't feel like patients here. . . . For a lot of us, the Center is like our family. . . . What's special about the Center is the sense of hope and the feeling of acceptance" (National League for Nursing, 1989).

In a letter written in 1990 by a client and signed by about 40 others, concern was expressed that as the DNPHC grows, the closeness and family-like environment may be diminished. The closing words of the letter are, "We welcome the growth of The Caring Center but hope it can proceed without losing the orientation to the clients that has made us love it and consider it a vital part of our lives." While this letter is both a tribute and a challenge to those of us responsible for guiding the DNPHC in its future development, the concern expressed in the letter can also lead to rich possibilities for study of this important environment.

History and Facility

The Denver Nursing Project in Human Caring opened in July 1988 as a nurse-directed outpatient facility designed to serve HIV positive/AIDS clients. The idea for the project originated during conversations between nurse administrators at two Denver hospitals—Denver Veterans Administration Medical Center (DVAMC) and Denver General Hospital (DGH)—who were concerned that the needs of this client population were being inadequately met in their respective facilities. Soon representatives of the University of Colorado School of Nursing Center for Human Caring were invited to participate in deliberations to find a way to deliver humanistic, holistic, individualized, and caring services. Later, nurses from the University of Colorado Hospital also became involved.

A descriptive "tour" of DNPHC begins as one steps into the 2,340-square-foot building that houses the facility located on the campus of the DVAMC. (The space has been donated since the beginning of the project.) This rectangular building consists of a long central hallway with rooms on each side, each with many windows. There are bright paintings and framed posters throughout the building and plenty of bulletin boards for displaying pertinent information. There are also always bouquets of fresh flowers in every room, donated weekly by the floral department of a local supermarket and arranged by a client volunteer.

A small entry room allows space for clients to sign in each time they visit the facility and indicate the services for which they have come. The office nearby is used for scheduling, record-keeping, and clerical necessities.

The large room just beyond the entry doubles as a treatment room and the kitchen area. Medical treatments include blood transfusions, IVs, chemotherapy, skin testing, drawing blood for lab work, and teaching self-care for some of these activities. The next major room in the building is the living room. It includes comfortable furnishings, a wonderful old upright piano, and a table that always has snacks, tea, and coffee. Every Friday, a complimentary lunch (furnished by local restaurants, organizations, and individual donations) is available to clients and visitors to the Center.

A little further down the hallway are two smaller rooms. The one on the left is the meditation room. Its healthy goldfish and taped music provide a comforting environment for "just being there." This room is also used by several massage therapists who provide services to clients every day of the week, using the portable massage table that was donated when DNPHC opened. Across the hall is a treatment room where medical treatments are given. Finally, there are two larger rooms that function as the education room and the support group room.

Programs and Services

The brochure for DNPHC categorizes services into three basic areas: medical/physical, educational, and psychosocial/emotional. In addition to the medical-dependent procedures described above, the first category includes nursing assessment of physical status of clients, appropriate referrals, and education to facilitate physical self-care. (An aerobics program and a cooperative arrangement with the University of Colorado School of Dentistry to provide dental screenings are currently very popular).

Educational services are offered in both individual and group formats. Attention is given to including content relevant to the disease process; updates in drug and treatment opportunities; and orientation to alternative healing modalities including meditation, visualization, therapeutic touch, nutritional information, and yoga.

Psychosocial/emotional services include numerous support groups, referral for individual counseling, referral for social service assistance, referral to other AIDS service organizations, periodic spiritual guidance programs, and much one-on-one conversation between nurses and clients. The clients elect a client advisory committee to facilitate liaison between staff and clients.

Financial Base and Numbers of Clients Served

Thus far, the three hospitals mentioned and the University of Colorado School of Nursing have totally supported DNPHC by providing the salaries for the nursing personnel and the space for the facility. Nurse administrators from the three hospitals and Jean Watson of the Center for Human Caring at the University of Colorado School of Nursing meet regularly as advisors to the project.

Clients eligible for DNPHC services are those whose HIV positivity has been verified and whose primary medical care originates in one of the three cooperating hospitals. Charges for supplies necessary for medically ordered treatments are referred back to the respective institutions.

Clerical work and building maintenance have been accomplished through cooperation of the nursing personnel and volunteers (both laypersons and clients.) There have been many examples of generous community support by donation of money and equipment such as microwave ovens, design and printing of brochures and stationery, an air compressor, televisions, and videocassette recorders. (Following a newspaper report of a robbery in the building earlier this year, voluntary replacement of everything lost plus additional items occurred within eight hours!)

Since the project opened, the total number of client visits is over 4,200. (This represents total visits during the 26 hours per week the DNPHC is open.) The current number of individuals being served at least once per month is nearly 100. The number of visits per month has increased steadily.

The Future

The cooperative arrangement among the sponsoring agencies will continue into the foreseeable future augmented by several factors. DNPHC has been awarded three grants during the past year. The first, from Aetna Life Insurance Company, is facilitating the production of a videotape about the project to be used in the hospitals and clinics from which clients come.

The second grant, from the Insurance Industry AIDS Initiative, provides salary for a part-time nurse to coordinate a Peer Assistance Program in which clients will be grouped with four or five other clients and a lay volunteer into "caring units." It is anticipated that by providing structure to such small groups, clients will have the opportunity to learn and grow from personal caring commitments as well as feel "permitted" to be cared for by others as their health needs dictate. The assessment and evaluation documents being developed for this project will provide meaningful information about clients' expectations regarding caring and their experiences as care providers for one another.

The third and most significant grant has been approved by the Department of Health and Human Services' Division of Nursing. Funding is anticipated beginning in summer 1990 and will continue for three years. The grant will allow the hiring of additional personnel to expand programs, provide more consistent case management, and conduct research relevant to caring theory. It will also make it possible to investigate and evaluate the feasibility, accountability, and appropriateness of the caring model within the health care environment.

CONCLUSION

Caring is "holding up the arc" to provide an enhanced quality of life for AIDS/HIV clients at the Denver Nursing Project. As Dr. Rieux found during the plague, the "common humanity" of clients and caregivers provides the basis for companionship, empathy, and mutual empowerment as persons progressing along life's journey. Emmanuel (Rodegast & Stanton, 1987) said he sees human beings as rainbows when he views them with love. There are many rainbows at the Denver Nursing Project in Human Caring.

REFERENCES

Benner, P. (1984). *From novice to expert.* Menlo Park, CA: Addison-Wesley Publishing Co.

Campbell, A. V. (1984). *Professional care: Its meaning and practice.* Philadelphia: Fortress Press.

Camus, A. (1972). *The plague.* New York: Vintage Books.

Department of Health and Human Services, Public Health Service, Centers for Disease Control. (1990, February). *HIV/AIDS Surveillance, 39,* (7).

Huch, M. H. (1988). Theory-based practice: Structuring nursing care. *Nursing Science Quarterly, 1*(1), 6–7.

Jones, A. H. (1990). Metaphors, narratives, and images of AIDS. *Medical Humanities Review, 4*(1), 7–16.

National League for Nursing. (1989). *Theories at work,* (Videotape). New York: Author.

Rodegast, P. & Stanton, J. (1987). *Emmanuel's book.* New York: Bantam Books.

Staff-(1989). *Mission Statement of the Denver Nursing Project in Human Caring.* Denver Nursing Project in Human Caring: Denver, CO.

Viney, L. L. (1983). *Images of illness.* Malabar, FL: Robert E. Krieger Publishing Co.

Watson, J. (1985a). *Nursing: The philosophy and science of caring.* Boulder, CO: Colorado Associated University Press.

Watson, J. (1985b). *Nursing: Human science and human care.* Norwalk, CT: Appleton-Century-Crofts.

Watson, J. (1987). Nursing on the caring edge: Metaphorical vignettes. *Advances in Nursing Science, 10*(1), 10–18.

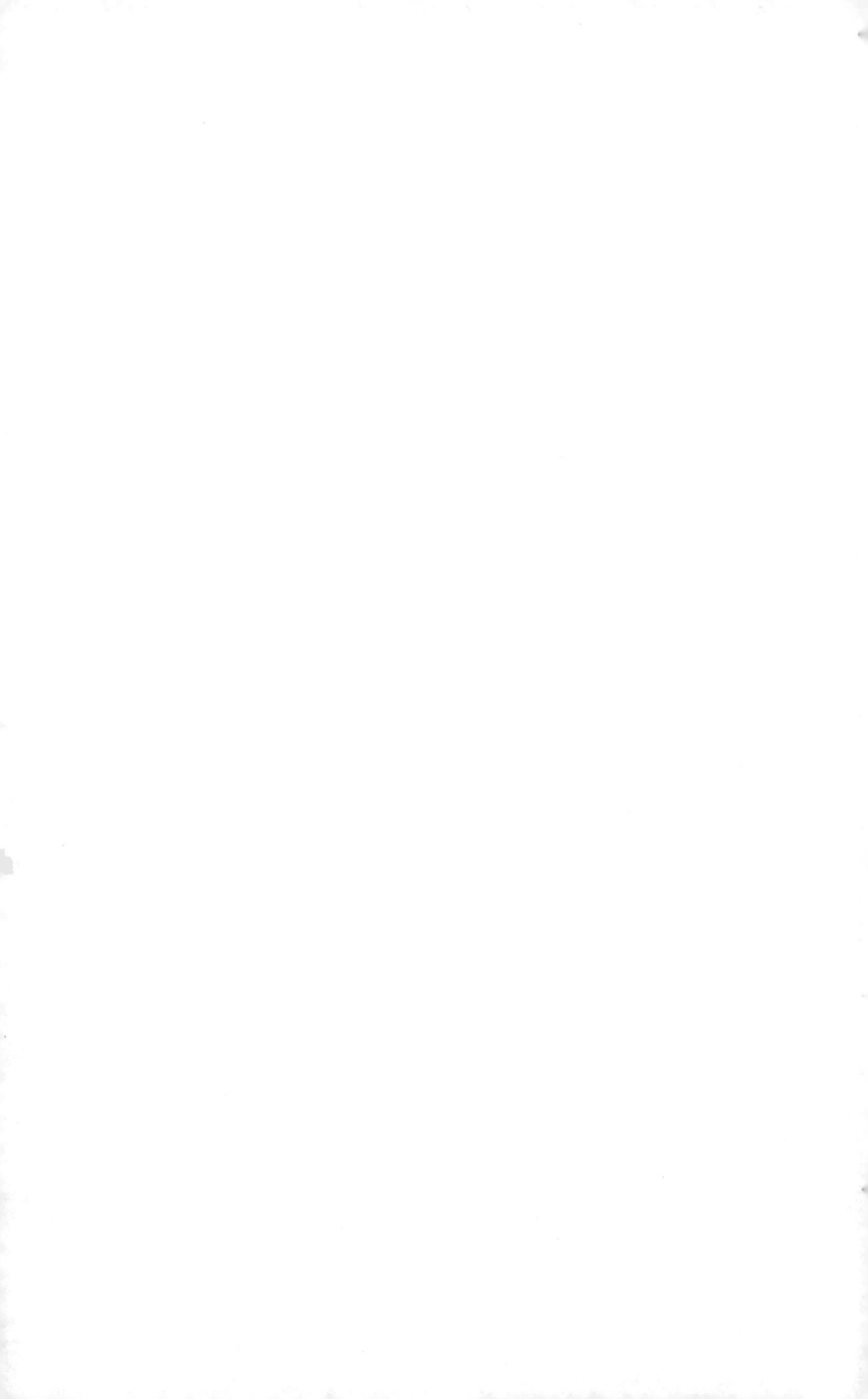

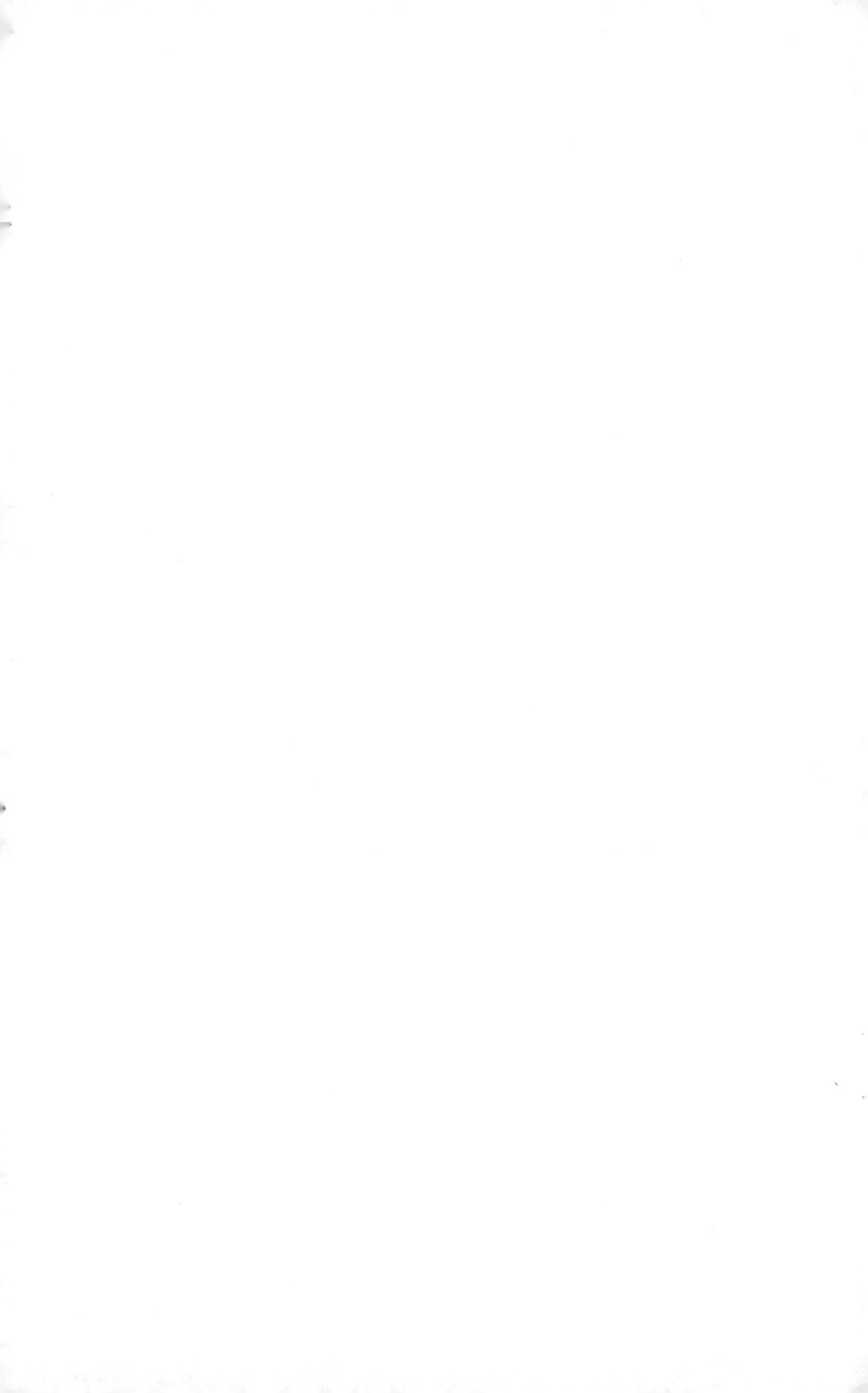